THE FITNESS INSTRUCTOR'S HANDBOOK

4TH EDITION

FITNESS
PROFESSIONALS

THE FITNESS INSTRUCTOR'S HANDBOOK

The Complete Guide to Health and Fitness

BLOOMSBURY SPORT

LONDON · OXFORD · NEW YORK · NEW DELHI · SYDNEY

MORC COULSON

BLOOMSBURY SPORT
Bloomsbury Publishing Plc
50 Bedford Square, London, WC1B 3DP, UK
29 Earlsfort Terrace, Dublin 2, Ireland

BLOOMSBURY, BLOOMSBURY SPORT and the Diana
logo are trademarks of Bloomsbury Publishing Plc

First published in Great Britain 2008, second edition,
2013, third edition, 2017
This edition published 2021

Copyright © Morc Coulson 2021
Inside photography courtesy of Grant Pritchard, Chris
Heron and David James Wood
Illustrations by Jeff Edwards and Dave Gardner

Morc Coulson has asserted his right under the
Copyright, Designs and Patents Act, 1988, to be
identified as Author of this work
For legal purposes the Acknowledgements on p. x
constitute an extension of this copyright page

Bloomsbury Publishing Plc does not have any control
over, or responsibility for, any third-party websites
referred to or in this book. All internet addresses given
in this book were correct at the time of going to press.
The author and publisher regret any inconvenience
caused if addresses have changed or sites have ceased
to exist, but can accept no responsibility for any such
changes

The information contained in this book is provided
by way of general guidance in relation to the specific
subject matters addressed herein, but it is not a
substitute for specialist advice. It should not be relied
on for medical, health-care, pharmaceutical or other
professional advice on specific dietary or health needs.
This book is sold with the understanding that the
author and publisher are not engaged in rendering
medical, health or any other kind of personal or
professional services. The reader should consult a
competent medical or health professional before
adopting any of the suggestions in this book or
drawing inferences from it. The author and publisher
specifically disclaim, as far as the law allows, any
responsibility from any liability, loss or risk (personal
or otherwise) which is incurred as a consequence,
directly or indirectly, of the use and applications of any
of the contents of this book.

Figure 11.2 is reprinted with permission from the
PAR-Q+ Collaboration (www.eparmedx.com) and
the authors of the PAR-Q+ (Dr. Darren Warburton,
Dr. Norman Gledhill, Dr. Veronica Jamnik, Dr. Roy
Shephard, and Dr. Shannon Bredin).

A catalogue record for this book is available from the
British Library

Library of Congress Cataloguing-in-Publication data
has been applied for

ISBN: PB: 978-1-4729-7734-2; eBook: 978-1-4729-7733-5

2 4 6 8 10 9 7 5 3 1

Typeset in Caecilia by Deanta Global Publishing
Services, Chennai, India
Printed and bound in Great Britain by CPI Group (UK)
Ltd., Croydon, CR0 4YY

To find out more about our authors and books visit
www.bloomsbury.com and sign up for our newsletters

CONTENTS

FOREWORD

Knowledge and support have helped many a top athlete over the years, not just physiologically but from a psychological, rehabilitational and medical perspective. It is common for individual athletes to use specifically designed programmes to train at the correct intensity, in the correct frame of mind and with nutritional advice that enables optimum recovery. There are also many recreational health and fitness participants who could benefit in many ways from support given by suitably qualified people. *The Fitness Instructor's Handbook* offers a comprehensive guide to the theory and practical application of health and fitness knowledge, linked closely to national occupational standards in this area. It is hoped that this book might help to develop a culture of education in health and fitness, not just for the benefit of the coach or instructor but for the entire population.

Steve Cram MBE and former BBC TV
Sports Personality of the Year

ACKNOWLEDGEMENTS

I would like to sincerely thank all who contributed in any way to the development and writing of this book including the editors at Bloomsbury. A big thank you goes out to the many instructors who continue to create an industry in which professionalism, passion and continuing personal development are considered as key attributes.

PREFACE

This book has been written for a wide audience, such as those who have an interest in health, fitness and sport, or as a reference guide for individuals who, both now and in the future, may be involved in prescribing gym-based cardiovascular and resistance exercise to clients who are referred to as 'apparently healthy'. The main objective of the book is to address the underpinning knowledge requirement related to gym qualifications in the health and fitness industry, and show how that knowledge can be applied in a practical environment. It was a conscious decision to relate the book to health and fitness qualification requirements for two main reasons: first, to provide a comprehensive textbook that could help promote the professionalism of the industry and second, to provide a text that covers comprehensively specific health and fitness knowledge criteria that are related to professional standards.

The chapter topics have been selected to provide a complete coverage of the required core knowledge content for Gym Instructor and Personal Trainer qualifications. At the end of the chapter you will find revision questions relating only to that particular chapter. Answers to these can be found at the back of the book, with space for revision notes. Each chapter also contains a list of further reading for those who would like to pursue the topic in more depth.

INTRODUCTION

Since 2003, the government has been committed to the development of the nation's skills and in particular the education and training provision to address the nation's skills gaps and shortages. In order to facilitate this intention, organisations such as the Fitness Industry Association (FIA), UK Active, SkillsActive and The Chartered Institute for the Management of Sport and Physical Activity (CIMSPA) have taken a lead role.

The FIA was founded in 1991 to drive up participation and address concerns in the industry relating to safety and unfair codes of conduct. In 2012 the FIA rebranded as UK Active. The fitness industry has since evolved and matured and, as the representative industry body, UK Active now works closely with government to help deliver its public health targets and represent the interests of more than 2500 health and fitness organisations across the United Kingdom. UK Active members include operators from the public and private sector, service/product suppliers to the industry, training providers, independent professionals and affiliated bodies. Members receive a variety of tailored, business-enhancing products and services specifically designed to support their particular business model or work.

UK Active's primary goal is to get more people more active, more often. This is primarily achieved by developing and running high-profile programmes designed to encourage people who are not regularly active to visit members' facilities.

SkillsActive was licensed by government as the Sector Skills Council for Active Leisure and Learning. Charged by employers, SkillsActive led the skills and productivity drive across the sport and recreation, health and fitness, outdoors, play work, and caravan industries – known as the active leisure and learning sector.

SkillsActive worked with health and fitness professionals across the United Kingdom to ensure the workforce was appropriately skilled and qualified. This included working with higher and further education to develop qualification frameworks for new qualifications to enable graduates to leave college or university with industry-recognised vocational qualifications. The Register of Exercise Professionals (REPs) was launched in 2002 as an independent, public register for the Health and Fitness Industry in the UK. Since 2016 REPs has been under the ownership of UK Coaching and in 2020 combined with the CIMSPA Exercise and Fitness directory to create a single register for all exercise fitness professionals. The intention of the register is to provide assurance and confidence to the public and employers alike that all professionals on the register are appropriately qualified and have the knowledge, competence and skills to perform their role effectively. This is essentially a process of self-regulation that recognises industry-based qualifications, practical competency, and requires fitness professionals to work to a Code of Ethical Practice within the framework of Professional Standards (these have replaced the National Occupational Standards that were developed by SkillsActive). Qualifications needed to gain entry to the directory are aligned with Professional Standards.

Duty of care (law of tort in England or delict in Scotland)

Any instructor working in the industry must be aware that they have a duty of care towards all individuals in that they must exercise a reasonable level of care in order to avoid injury to individuals and their property. In cases where breach of duty of care has been alleged it is the responsibility of the instructor to demonstrate that they have not acted in a negligent manner (a negligent act can be described as an unintentional but careless act that results in injury to a person or loss of property). This includes a duty of care towards vulnerable adults or clients that instructors are qualified to work with.

Note: A vulnerable adult is defined by the UK government as 'a person aged 18 years or over who is or may be in need of community care services by reason of mental or other disability, age or illness; and who is or may be unable to take care of themselves, or unable to protect themselves against significant harm or exploitation'. A vulnerable client is someone undergoing a 'special' physiological lifespan process that puts them at a greater risk of an exercise-related event (e.g. childhood, ageing, ante- and post-natal).

THEORETICAL KNOWLEDGE
FOR HEALTH AND FITNESS

Part 1 of this book addresses the theoretical knowledge required for instructors within the Health and Fitness Industry. Each chapter provides example questions that are typical of Industry Standard questions provided by accredited centres for the delivery of recognised qualifications. Part 1 also provides a list of recommended reading for each chapter, should the reader wish to gain a more in-depth knowledge of the relevant topic area.

1 The Skeletal System

OBJECTIVES

After completing this chapter, you will be able to:

1 Describe the structure of bone, in particular long bones.
2 Classify bones and give examples of each type.
3 Describe the process of bone growth, in particular within long bones.
4 Discuss the factors that can affect bone density.
5 Explain the effects of exercise on bone.
6 Describe the structure and list the functions of the skeleton.
7 Identify the major bones in the body.
8 Describe the structure and list the functions of the vertebral column.
9 Describe the structure and function of vertebral and intervertebral discs.
10 Describe the range of motion available at the spine.
11 Describe common postural definitions and list a range of common injuries associated with the spine.

Introduction

This chapter deals with the anatomical systems of the body, in particular the formation of bone and the skeletal system from the perspective of structure and function, as well as the effects of exercise on these systems. Within the Professional Standards framework, instructors should be able to identify the components of the skeletal system and describe their functions, as well as describe how exercise can impact on bone growth.

Later chapters provide physiological and biomechanical principles that, together with the anatomical knowledge covered in this chapter, will provide fitness instructors with the understanding and ability to design appropriate exercise programmes for apparently healthy individuals and to understand the effects of various types of exercise on the human body.

Common anatomical terms

As the first part of this book is concerned with the anatomy of the human body, it is useful to understand the terms used to describe it. When

TABLE 1.1

Common anatomical terms

Term	Description
Anterior	Front
Posterior	Back
Medial	Towards the midline
Lateral	Away from the midline
Superior	Upper
Inferior	Lower
Proximal	Near to
Distal	Away from
Prone	Facing down
Supine	Facing up

using anatomical terms, the body is assumed to be in a position where the arms are resting by the sides of the body with the palms facing forward, with a theoretical line drawn down the centre of the body. When the limbs move, the movement is described in reference to this line. Table 1.1 contains some common anatomical terms and their description.

Bone

BONE STRUCTURE

Bone is classified as a calcified connective tissue and, when it is fully developed, is the hardest tissue in the body. In a typical bone there are two types of bone tissue: *compact* and *cancellous*.

• **Compact bone**   Compact bone is also known as *cortical* bone. It has a hard outer layer that provides a strong structure called the *cortex*, which provides protection and support to help resist stresses imposed during movement and weight-bearing activities. It is often assumed that compact bone is solid, but this is not the case: it contains a series of canals through which blood and lymph vessels and nerves pass. This series of canals gives compact bone greater strength than if the bone was completely solid, as the canal systems are aligned in the same direction along the lines of stress of each bone, helping to resist fracture.

• **Cancellous bone**   Cancellous bone is otherwise known as *trabecular* bone. Within cancellous bone there is a 'spongy' structure that contains red bone marrow, which is where blood cells are made. This type of bone also contains a series of canals that are larger than those in compact bone as the red bone marrow needs to get a rich blood supply to produce red blood cells.

A double layer of tough, dense collagen fibres about the thickness of a nail, called the *periosteum*, covers most of the surface of bones. It provides attachment for tendons and ligaments and gives protection to the bone.

CLASSIFICATION OF BONES

Bones are often classified according to their formation and shape. The shape of a bone can sometimes help to identify the role it has in the body. Bone is normally classified into the five groups below (see also Fig. 1.1).

1 Long bones   Long bones are found mainly in the limbs and comprise a shaft with two extremities. The shaft is known as the

FIG. 1.1

Examples of the different types of bone in the body

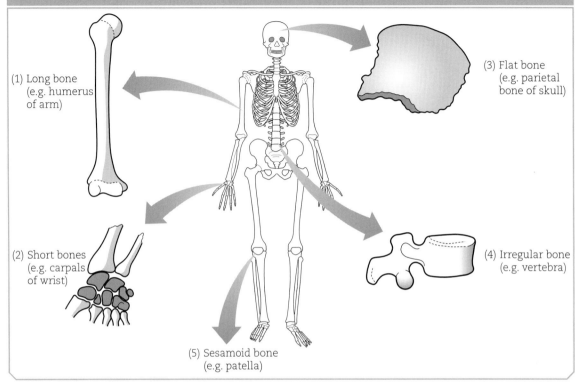

(1) Long bone
(e.g. humerus
of arm)

(3) Flat bone
(e.g. parietal
bone of skull)

(2) Short bones
(e.g. carpals
of wrist)

(4) Irregular bone
(e.g. vertebra)

(5) Sesamoid bone
(e.g. patella)

diaphysis and the extremities are known as the *epiphyses*. Just before each epiphysis is a region known as the growth plate or *epiphyseal cartilage*. This is the region of the bone at which growth occurs; when growth finally stops in adulthood the epiphyseal cartilage becomes fully developed bone. Fatty yellow bone marrow is found within the central part of the long bone known as the *medullary canal*. Long bones are attached to muscles that can pull and create movement, so they act as levers to provide locomotion for the body. The femur and humerus are examples of long bones.

2 Short bones Short bones are designed mainly for lightness and strength. They are usually cube-shaped and are mainly spongy (cancellous) bone with a thin outer layer of compact bone. Examples of short bones are the carpals (wrist) and tarsals (ankle).

3 Flat bones Flat bones are spongy (cancellous) bones sandwiched between two layers of compact bone. They either give protection, such as in the skull, or provide a large area for muscle attachment, such as in the pelvis.

4 Irregular bones Irregular bones usually have bony projections for the purpose of muscle attachment. The vertebrae (bones of the spine) are examples of irregular bones.

5 Sesamoid bones Sesamoid bones are seed-like bones, normally the size of a pea, that are developed within the tendon of a muscle, such as the patella in the knee joint. Sesamoid bones usually protect tendons from excessive wear and tear. They can also change the direction of pull of a tendon to increase the mechanical advantage at a joint in which the tendon crosses.

TASK
Fig. 1.1 shows examples of the five types of bone and where they can be found in the body. Try to identify all of the bones in the skeleton and assign them to one of the five classifications.

BONE GROWTH

Bone growth in humans begins at birth and is usually not complete until about the 25th year but can, in some cases, be complete around the age of 18. Bones start out in the body as tissues known as cartilage, membrane and tendon until a process called *ossification* (*oss* meaning bone and *fication* meaning to make) gradually replaces these tissues with bone. Certain hormones released within the body, such as growth hormone, testosterone, oestrogen and calcitonin, help to regulate and control bone development.

Long bones, such as those in the limbs, grow in length at the epiphyseal or growth plate, which is the region near the end of the diaphysis or shaft of the bone (see Fig. 1.2). The ends, or epiphyses, of long bones are enlarged and are

FIG. 1.2

The structure of a typical long bone

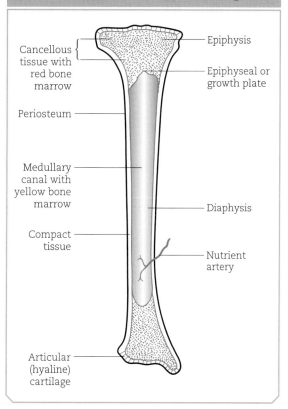

Cancellous tissue with red bone marrow

Epiphysis

Epiphyseal or growth plate

Periosteum

Medullary canal with yellow bone marrow

Diaphysis

Compact tissue

Nutrient artery

Articular (hyaline) cartilage

covered in a tissue called hyaline cartilage (see page 67), which provides protection for the end of the bone.

TASK
Draw and label the parts of a typical long bone and list the functions of each part.

Bone tissue contains several types of cell. An *osteocyte* is the main cell of a fully developed bone. Two other types of bone cell, *osteoblasts* and *osteoclasts*, are responsible for building and modelling the bone in which they are located. Osteoblasts are bone-building cells that are involved in the formation of bone; osteoclasts are very large bone-modelling cells that can break down bone formation by digesting protein and minerals, making the bone less dense and therefore weaker. Throughout life, if homeostasis is achieved, then osteoblasts and osteoclasts work together to keep bone at the optimum thickness. If homeostasis is disrupted, it is possible that one type of bone cell can dominate, resulting in either a thickening or weakening of the bone.

Ossification can start as early as in the womb, where osteoblasts secrete protein (primarily collagen) to initiate the process of calcification by forming a meshwork called the *bone matrix*. Osteoblasts get trapped in the matrix and become osteocytes (main bone cells) as the matrix calcifies and hardens. Other osteoblasts then work outwards to increase the length of the bone. At the same time, osteoclasts work to remove excess bone and prevent it from becoming too thick. Osteoblasts and osteoclasts work together at the epiphyses of the bone to form an epiphyseal plate, which is responsible for bone growth. This activity is controlled by many hormones at different stages throughout life; one of the most important is growth hormone, which is secreted by the *pituitary gland*. As a result growth spurts can occur at different times, typically at the ages of 10–13 for girls and 12–14 for boys. During growth, the epiphyseal plate is just a layer of hyaline cartilage. When bones stop growing in length (usually between the ages of 18 and 25) the hyaline cartilage at the epiphyseal plate is replaced by bone. Even though bones do not grow in length after this stage, they can continue to grow in diameter throughout life.

NEED TO KNOW
Other hormones that influence bone growth include thyroxine, testosterone, oestrogen, calcitonin and parathormone.

• Factors affecting bone growth

Age, lack of weight-bearing activity, smoking and alcoholism can all lead to a loss of calcium and bone marrow. The cancellous part of the bone, therefore, becomes less dense, making the bone weaker and slower to heal. A severe case of this condition is known as osteoporosis, which is more common in females (especially post-menopausal) than males: figures suggest that up to 50 per cent of post-menopausal women suffer from the condition. Even though it is thought that osteoporosis is not reversible, many studies have shown that exercise can slow down the rate at which osteoporosis occurs – the pull of muscles on bone and the effects of gravity can lead to an increase in bone density (Baechle, 2016; Kenney, Wilmore and Costhill, 2019). It is therefore important that some type of resistance training be recommended to people with this condition, although care should be taken due to the risk of bone fracture or breaks.

NEED TO KNOW
The density of bone can be estimated using a technique known as dual-energy X-ray absorptiometry (DEXA). This technique, which involves a very low dose of photon radiation, can also be used to estimate body-fat percentage.

Diet also has an impact on bone growth and strength. Almost half the content of bone is made up of the minerals calcium and phosphorus. Calcium is always present in the blood as it has many functions in the body; for example, it is required for muscle contraction and bone formation (normal blood calcium levels are 9–11mg per 100ml of blood). If blood calcium levels fall, osteoclasts will break down bone to release calcium into the bloodstream. Therefore, a diet low in calcium can make the bones weaker. About 80 per cent of the phosphorus in the body is found in and is responsible for the formation of bones and teeth. It also plays an important part in muscle contraction. Dietary sources include dairy products, meat, fish and beans. Finally, vitamins C and D are also important in the process of bone growth: vitamin C is used in the laying down of collagen to form connective tissue, such as in bone formation, while vitamin D is essential for the absorption of calcium and phosphorus from the intestine.

The effects of exercise on bone

Physical activity has been shown to stimulate osteoblasts to secrete protein and initiate the bone-building process as a result of placing force on the bone. This is referred to as the *minimal essential strain*. The exact amount of activity required to start this process is unknown, but is thought to be equivalent to one-tenth of the force required to fracture the bone. Forces placed on the bone below this threshold are believed to have no effect. Many studies have also shown a correlation between bone density and the strength of the attached musculature, so it appears that resistance training has a positive effect on bone density. However, the formation of new bone is relatively slow compared to the rapid loss of bone mineral content as a result of immobility or reduced loading, especially following a period of bed-rest.

NEED TO KNOW

In general terms, an increase or decrease in muscle strength will result in a corresponding increase or decrease in bone density.

SHORT-TERM EFFECTS

There are no actual short-term effects of exercise on the bones; instead, exercise initiates the long-term process described below.

LONG-TERM EFFECTS

Placing stress on the bones by engaging in weight-bearing exercise is thought to result in the bone tissue becoming stronger over a period of time. However, care must be taken not to place too much stress or high impact on the bones of children who have not fully matured, as this can result in damage to the epiphyseal plate or other injuries such as Chondromalacia patellae, Osgood-Schlatter disease and Sever's disease.

Exactly how placing stress on the bones results in stronger bone tissue is still a case for debate. However, it is commonly agreed that resistance or impact exercise places stress on the bones that stimulate this mechanism. It is recommended that adolescents and young adults should engage in some sort of weight-bearing activity to help this process occur, but, as stated above, the amount of stress must be limited.

It is also recommended that older adults engage in some sort of bone-stressing exercise, because as we get older the amount of calcium taken out of the bones is greater than the amount of calcium taken in by the bones. This is due to the fact that activity levels and dietary intake of calcium and phosphorus usually reduces, while in post-menopausal women a reduction in hormone levels disrupts the activity of osteoblasts. In the long term, this makes the bones less dense and therefore weaker.

NEED TO KNOW
Astronauts in space can lose as much as 1 per cent of bone mass per week due to the lack of gravity.

The skeleton

STRUCTURE AND FUNCTIONS OF THE SKELETON

The human skeleton contains approximately 206 bones and consists of two parts: the *axial skeleton*, which comprises the skull, the vertebral column (backbone), the ribs and the sternum; and the *appendicular skeleton* (*appendic* meaning 'to hang on to'), which comprises the shoulder and pelvic girdles and the upper and lower limbs (see Fig. 1.3). The skeleton as a whole has many important functions, including:

- Providing a framework and shape for the body: the size and shape of the skeleton can determine a person's shape (see page 159).
- Protecting the vital organs: for example, the ribcage protects the heart and lungs.
- Acting as levers for movement on which muscles act. When muscles contract they draw together and, as the ends of muscles are normally attached to bones, one attachment will move towards the other.
- Providing surfaces for the attachment of muscles (via tendons) and ligaments.
- Producing red and white blood cells and platelets. This is the function of the cancellous or 'spongy' bone.
- Storing minerals such as calcium, phosphorus, potassium and sodium.

It is important that health and fitness instructors are familiar with the names and locations of the bones in the body as, together with the muscles, they provide movement and locomotion.

- **The bones of the shoulder (pectoral) girdle** See Table 1.2 and Fig. 1.4. The shoulder or pectoral girdle attaches the arms to the body, or, in other words, the upper limbs to the axial skeleton. It consists of a *scapula* (shoulder blade) and *clavicle* (collarbone) on each side of the body. The scapula has a socket called the *glenoid fossa* or *cavity*, which articulates (joins) with the upper arm (*humerus*) to form the shoulder joint. This is a shallow joint that allows for a large degree of mobility at the expense of stability. The most lateral point of the scapula is called the *acromion process*, which articulates with the clavicle to form the acromioclavicular joint. The distance between the two acromion processes is called the *biacromial distance*.

- **The bones of the upper and lower arm** See Table 1.3 and Fig. 1.5. The humerus is the bone of the upper arm that, along with the glenoid fossa of the scapula, makes the shoulder joint. The distal (far) end of the humerus articulates with the two bones of the lower arm or forearm (with the *radius* at the *capitulum* and with the *ulna* at the *trochlea*) to form the elbow joint.

- **The bones of the hand and wrist** See Table 1.4 and Fig. 1.6. The eight short bones located in the wrist are known collectively as the *carpals*. The bones are held together tightly by ligaments (see pages 67 and 70) and have only a small degree of movement. The carpal bones articulate with the ulna and radius to form the wrist joint. At their furthest point, the carpals articulate with five bones

FIG. 1.3

The bones of (a) the axial and (b) the appendicular skeleton

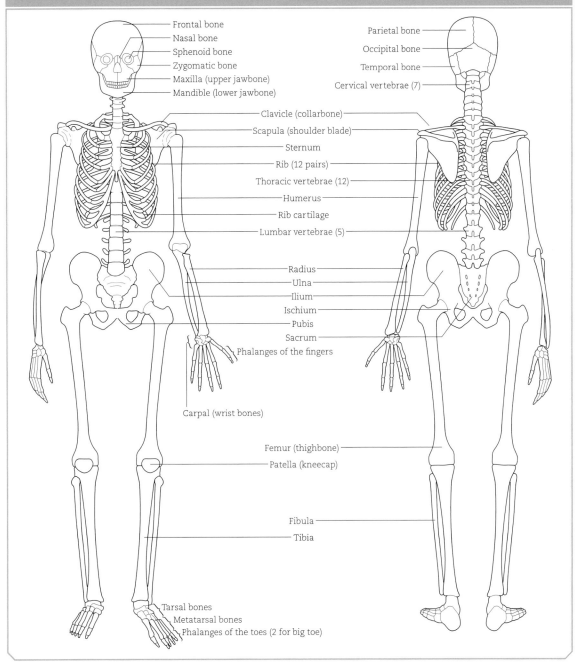

Frontal bone
Nasal bone
Sphenoid bone
Zygomatic bone
Maxilla (upper jawbone)
Mandible (lower jawbone)

Parietal bone
Occipital bone
Temporal bone
Cervical vertebrae (7)

Clavicle (collarbone)
Scapula (shoulder blade)
Sternum
Rib (12 pairs)
Thoracic vertebrae (12)
Humerus
Rib cartilage
Lumbar vertebrae (5)

Radius
Ulna
Ilium
Ischium
Pubis
Sacrum
Phalanges of the fingers

Carpal (wrist bones)

Femur (thighbone)
Patella (kneecap)

Fibula
Tibia

Tarsal bones
Metatarsal bones
Phalanges of the toes (2 for big toe)

TABLE 1.2

The bones of the shoulder girdle

Bone	Landmark	Description
Scapula	Acromion process	Projection over the shoulder joint Site of muscular attachment Articulates with the clavicle
	Coracoid process	Projection on the anterior aspect of the scapula Site of attachment for the short head of the biceps
	Spine of the scapula	Large ridge extending from the acromion process across the posterior surface of the scapula to the medial border of the scapula
	Glenoid fossa	Shallow depression where the humerus articulates with the scapula
Clavicle	Acromial end	Articulates with the acromion process of the scapula
	Sternal end	Articulates with the manubrium of the sternum

FIG. 1.4

Bones of the shoulder girdle

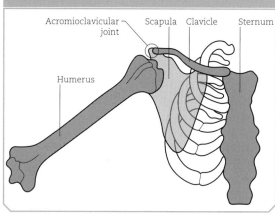

in the palm of the hand called the *metacarpals* (*meta* meaning 'beyond'). The metacarpals then articulate with the fingers or *phalanges*, each of which comprises proximal (near), medial (middle) and distal (far) sections, except for the thumb, which has only two sections.

• The bones of the pelvic girdle
See Table 1.5 and Fig. 1.7. The pelvic girdle provides a strong base to which the axial skeleton attaches via the vertebral column, making a fused joint with the *sacrum*. This is called the *sacroiliac joint*. On each side of the pelvis is a socket called the *acetabulum*, which forms a joint with the femur of the upper leg. This is a deep socket that provides a high degree of stability, but has less mobility than

TABLE 1.3

The bones of the upper and lower arm

Bone	Landmark	Description
Humerus	Head	Smooth, round proximal surface that articulates with the glenoid fossa of the scapula
	Humeral condyles (capitulum and trochlea)	Articular surfaces on the medial and lateral sides of the distal humerus Capitulum articulates with the head of the radius Trochlea articulates with the trochlear notch on the ulna
Ulna	Olecranon process	Process at the proximal end of the ulna Point of the elbow Attachment point for the posterior arm muscles
	Head	Small, partially rounded distal end that articulates with the radius and wrist bones
Radius	Head	Proximal, drum-shaped end Articulates with the capitulum of the humerus and the radial notch of the ulna

the shoulder girdle. The pelvic girdle protects the internal organs, and in women also provides protection for the foetus during pregnancy. The distance between the two most lateral points is known as the *bicristal distance* and is usually greater in females than in males.

• The bones of the upper and lower leg See Table 1.6 and Fig. 1.8. The *femur* (thigh bone) is a long bone in the upper leg and is the longest bone in the body. At the top or head of the femur is a ball-shaped part of the bone that articulates with the socket (*acetabulum*) of the pelvis to form the hip joint. At the bottom of the femur are two smooth, rounded surfaces that articulate with the *tibia* to form the *tibiofemoral* or knee joint. Each end

of the femur is covered in hyaline cartilage (see page 67).

At the front of the knee joint is a small, triangular sesamoid bone called the *patella* (meaning 'little dish'), which is otherwise known as the kneecap. The patella is located within a band of tendon (see page 39) and glides over the groove on the end of the femur as the knee joint flexes and extends. This is known as the *patellofemoral joint*.

The *tibia* is the main weight-bearing bone in the lower leg and is sometimes known as the shin bone. The top of the tibia is a broad flat surface that articulates with the femur to form the knee joint. The bottom of the tibia articulates with one of the tarsal bones in the ankle, called the *talus*, to form the ankle joint.

TABLE 1.4

The bones of the hand and wrist

Bone	Landmark	Description
Carpals	Triquetrum Trapezoid Trapezium Hamate Lunate Capitate Pisiform Scaphoid	Articulate with the radius and ulna at the proximal side and with the metacarpals at the distal side
Metacarpals		Short bones located within the palm
Phalanges	Proximal, medial and distal	Proximal, medial and distal sections allow individual movement for dexterity

FIG. 1.5

Upper and lower arm

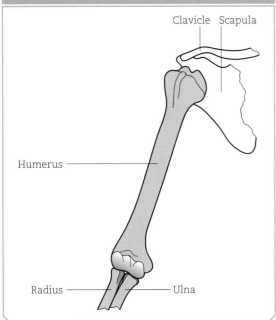

Clavicle Scapula

Humerus

Radius   Ulna

The *fibula* is a long bone that runs down the lateral side of the tibia and makes a fibrous joint (see pages 24 and 25) at both ends with the tibia.

• The bones of the foot and ankle

See Table 1.7 and Fig. 1.9. The seven short bones in the back section of the foot are collectively known as the *tarsals*. The *calcaneus* is the largest of the tarsal bones and is otherwise known as the heel bone. The *talus* is most superior and articulates with the tibia to form the ankle joint. As with the carpals, the tarsal bones are held together tightly by ligaments (see pages 67 and 70) and have only a small degree of movement.

In the mid-foot are five bones known as the *metatarsals* that articulate with the toes, which, like the fingers, are known as *phalanges*. Again, like the fingers, each of the phalanges except for the big toe has three sections: the proximal (nearest), medial (middle) and distal (farthest) phalanges.

FIG. 1.6

Bones of the hand and the wrist

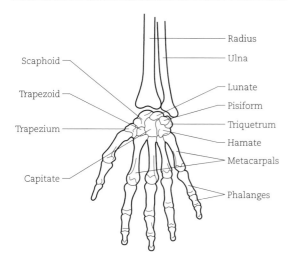

FIG. 1.7

Bones of the pelvic girdle

THE STRUCTURE AND FUNCTIONS OF THE VERTEBRAL COLUMN

The spine, otherwise known as the vertebral column or backbone, consists of 24 separate movable bones called *vertebrae* (separated by *intervertebral discs*) and nine fused bones. The movable bones are in three regions – *cervical*, *thoracic* and *lumbar* – and the fused bones are in two regions – *sacrum* and *coccyx* (see Fig. 1.10).

The spine is essentially a strong and flexible column that acts as a support system on which the limbs are able to move. Viewed from the side, the structure is curved. The thoracic and sacral regions of the spine are known as primary curves, while the cervical and lumbar regions are known as secondary curves. These curves increase the strength of the vertebral column and provide shock absorption during walking, running and jumping.

TABLE 1.5

The bones of the pelvic girdle

Bone	Landmark	Description
Ilium		Large, flat, superior wing-like portion of the pelvis
	Iliac crest	Large ridge on the superior part of the ilium
Ischium		Posterior, inferior portion of the pelvis
Pubis		Anterior, inferior portion of the pelvis
	Acetabulum	Depression into which the head of the femur articulates

FIG. 1.8

Bones of the upper and lower leg

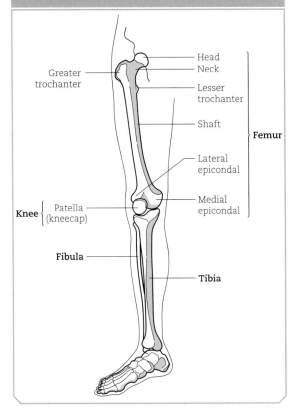

- Greater trochanter
- Head
- Neck
- Lesser trochanter
- Shaft
- **Femur**
- Lateral epicondal
- Medial epicondal
- **Knee**
- Patella (kneecap)
- **Fibula**
- **Tibia**

made up of five bones. There is a wide range of movement available in this region, as this is the part of the spine from which the upper body bends forward and from side to side. The region of the spine known as the sacrum consists of five fused bones and is attached to the pelvis. Finally, the coccyx at the bottom of the spine is made up of four fused bones, but really serves no purpose.

As well as attaching the lower part of the body to the upper part, the spine serves many other functions in the body, including:

- Protecting the spinal cord – the main nerve stem from the brain, which runs through a hole (*foramen*) in the posterior part of each vertebra
- Providing access for blood and lymph vessels
- Allowing certain degrees of movement – each individual vertebra does not have much movement, but the spine as a unit does
- Providing support for the skull
- Providing attachment for the ribs and pelvic girdle (the part of the vertebral bodies where the ribs attach to the spine is known as a *facet*)
- Housing shock-absorbing discs

The top vertebra in the spine is known as the *atlas* and makes a joint with the skull. The bone underneath the atlas is called the *axis* and, along with the atlas, provides a pivot that enables the skull to rotate. The neck region of the spine, made up of seven bones, is known as the cervical region and allows a degree of movement for the head. Below this, in the upper part of the body, is the thoracic region of the spine, which comprises 12 bones. Here, movement is limited as the ribcage is attached to the spine in this region. Below this, in the lower part of the back, is the lumbar spine,

VERTEBRAL BODIES AND INTERVERTEBRAL DISCS

The vertebrae in different regions of the spine can vary slightly in shape and size but essentially share the same features (see Fig. 1.11), especially between the second cervical vertebra and the fifth lumbar vertebra. Each vertebra has a disc-shaped body with several bony processes that extend from the back of the body, which allow for the attachment of muscles via tendons. At the ends of the bony processes are surfaces known as *facets* that are covered in smooth tissue called *articular*

TABLE 1.6

The bones of the upper and lower leg

Bone	Landmark	Description
Femur	Head	Articulates with the acetabulum of the pelvis
	Greater trochanter	Large process on the lateral side of the proximal end of the bone, to which the gluteal muscles attach
	Condyles	Rounded medial and lateral smooth articular surfaces where the femur articulates with the tibia
	Intercondylar fossa	Deep groove between the condyles where the cruciate ligaments attach
	Epicondyles	Small medial and lateral ridges where the muscles attach
Tibia	Condyles	Flat, smooth medial and lateral surfaces with which the femur articulates
	Intercondylar eminence	Crest between the condyles where the cruciate ligaments attach
	Tibial tuberosity	Knot on the anterior, proximal surface where the patellar ligament attaches
	Medial malleolus	Large process of the distal, medial aspect of the bone
Fibula	Head	Proximal enlargement Articulates with the lateral aspect of the proximal tibia
	Lateral malleolus	Enlargement on the distal, lateral aspect of the bone
Patella		Large sesamoid bone in the tendon of the quadriceps muscles of the anterior thigh

cartilage. The facets of one vertebra make a joint, known as a *zygapophyseal joint*, with the facets of the vertebrae above and below. These joints are synovial (gliding) joints – lubricated with synovial fluid – that allow movement of the spine. The range of motion in each section of the spine mainly depends on the facet joints. The main body of a typical vertebra has an opening

TABLE 1.7

The bones of the foot and ankle

Bone	Landmark	Description
Tarsals	Calcaneus talus Cuboid cuneiform (×3) Navicular	The talus articulates with the tibia and fibula at the proximal side The 3 cuneiform bones and the cuboid articulate with the metatarsals at the distal side
Metatarsals		Short bones located between the ankle joint and the mid-foot
Phalanges	Proximal, medial and distal	Proximal, medial and distal sections to allow individual movement and flexibility

on the posterior side known as a *vertebral foramen*, which provides a protective channel through which the spinal cord can run. Nerves branching out from the spinal cord exit from gaps between each adjacent pair of vertebrae.

Between the bodies of adjacent vertebrae are *intervertebral discs* (see Fig. 1.11), which provide shock absorption for the spine. The outer layer of the disc, called the *annulus fibrosus* (annulus meaning 'ring-like'), is made of cartilaginous fibres and is very tough. The inner part of the disc is called the *nucleus pulposus* (pulposus meaning 'pulp-like') and is made of a soft, viscous, fluid-like material that is very elastic.

Together with the vertebrae, the intervertebral discs provide strong joints in the spine that can withstand a certain amount of compression and stretching. However, it is possible for the outer layer of the disc (the annulus fibrosus) to be ruptured so that the inner part of the disc (the nucleus pulposus) protrudes. This is commonly known as a *slipped* or *herniated disc*. It is possible for the nucleus

pulposus to exert pressure on a spinal nerve, causing pain either locally or along the length of the nerve.

The discs increase in thickness from the top to the bottom of the spine and can reduce

FIG. 1.9

Bones of the foot and ankle

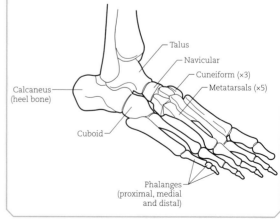

Talus
Navicular
Cuneiform (×3)
Metatarsals (×5)
Calcaneus (heel bone)
Cuboid
Phalanges (proximal, medial and distal)

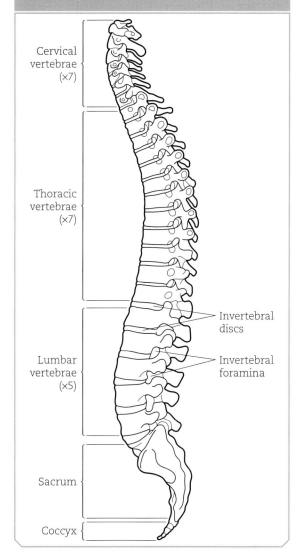

FIG. 1.10

The vertebral column

Cervical vertebrae (×7)

Thoracic vertebrae (×7)

Lumbar vertebrae (×5)

Invertebral discs

Invertebral foramina

Sacrum

Coccyx

Range of movement of the vertebral column

The range of movement between each individual bone in the spine is limited because of the facet joints, as mentioned above. However, the spine as a whole is capable of a wide range of movement, including *flexion* (bending forward), *extension* (bending backwards), *lateral flexion* or *extension* (bending to the side) and *rotation*. The spine has more movement in the cervical and lumbar regions than anywhere else. Flexion and extension of the spine occur mainly at the lower two lumbar vertebrae; however, there is a limited degree of rotation at the lumbar spine. Flexion and extension are limited in the thoracic spine due to the attachment of the ribs, but there is a reasonable amount of rotation.

Age can decrease the movement available in the spine; it is therefore recommended that mobilisation and flexibility exercises make up an important part of an overall exercise programme with older adults.

There are many published tables available that provide information about the ranges of motion available at the spine. However, the ranges of motion can differ depending on which author has published the tables; therefore, Table 1.8 shows a typical range of motion for movements of the spine that are common to the published ranges.

NEED TO KNOW

The secondary cervical curve develops only after about the first three months of life and the lumbar curve after 12 to 18 months.

in thickness throughout the day due to the effects of compression and lack of hydration. The discs can return to their original size overnight if hydrated, but due to the ageing process can degenerate and become thinner as we get older.

FIG. 1.11

A typical vertebral body

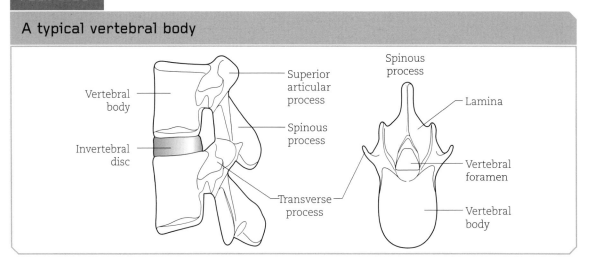

POSTURAL DEFINITIONS

The facet joints and intervertebral discs provide the spine with a certain amount of rigidity, but this is not an adequate amount of support to maintain posture at all times. The muscles provide a certain amount of support, as do the many ligaments that surround the spine (see Fig. 1.12). There are two main groups of ligaments related to the spine: the *intrasegmental* and the *intersegmental* ligaments. Like all ligaments, the spinal ligaments allow a certain degree of wanted movement, but are designed to prevent unwanted movement.

The small range of motion at the spine where none of the spinal ligaments are placed under any tension is known as the *neutral zone*. This is considered to be correct alignment or posture for the spine. Postural deviations can occur where spinal ligaments have been stretched, where spinal muscles are weak or where there are mechanical dysfunctions. Postural deviation is a general term used to describe any posture considered different

TABLE 1.8

Typical range of motion associated with the spinal column

Movement	Range of motion
Flexion	Total range of 45–55 degrees, mainly at the lumbar region
Extension	Typically 20–35 degrees
Lateral flexion	Up to 60 degrees to either side of the midline, but reducing quickly with age
Rotation	Limited to only a few degrees in the lumbar spine

FIG. 1.12

Typical spinous ligaments

Ligamentum flavum

Facet capsulary ligament

Interspinous ligament

Supraspinous ligament

Intertransverse ligament

Posterior longitudinal ligament

Anterior longitudinal ligament

to the 'norm'. There are many methods used to assess posture that typically use a plumb-line approach in which certain landmarks (on the shoulders, hips, knees and ankles for example) are compared for position and symmetry in relation to an 'ideal' posture. Common postural deviations include *kyphosis*, *lordosis* and *scoliosis*.

● **Kyphosis**   This term is used to describe an excessive secondary curve of the thoracic region of the spine. People who suffer from this condition are usually very round-shouldered or hunched in appearance. The diagnosis can often be complicated, but common back-strengthening exercises for the trapezius and rhomboid muscles are normally advocated.

Note: During pregnancy there is likely to be a greater forward shift of centre of gravity, which increases lordosis (curved lower back) and can contribute to kyphosis (rounded shoulders).

● **Lordosis**   This term describes an excessive primary curve of the lumbar region of the spine. The condition is sometimes referred to as 'swayback' and is often associated with an increase in abdominal weight, for example, in pregnancy or obesity. Core stabilisation techniques are usually prescribed, as the anterior spinal ligaments can be damaged by this type of posture.

● **Scoliosis**   There are different types of scoliosis, but the term generally refers to a twisting or abnormal curvature of the spine. Scoliosis is normally associated with the thoracic or upper lumbar areas of the spine, although in some cases it can occur in the lower part of the lumbar region. Specific exercises

TABLE 1.9

Types of scoliosis

Scoliosis type	Description
Congenital	This type of congenital deformity is quite rare
Neuromuscular	Due to muscle weakness or imbalance, it is possible for the spine to be pulled to one side
Degenerative	Due to the ageing process, it is possible for the spine to develop scoliosis
Idiopathic	This type of scoliosis normally develops in adolescence and usually has no known cause

are sometimes effective to rectify muscular imbalance, but these need to be prescribed by a qualified person. For the different types of scoliosis, see Table 1.9.

COMMON SPINAL INJURIES

The spine is a complex mechanical structure and is therefore susceptible to many possible injuries. Injuries can occur in relation to the vertebrae, the spinal ligaments, the intervertebral discs, the spinal muscle and tendons or associated spinal nerves.

• Vertebral body injuries

Fractures
Fractures to the vertebral body can be caused as a result of an external blow, known as an *extrinsic* injury, or as a result of internal forces, known as an *intrinsic* injury.

Spondylolysis
This term refers to the degenerative destruction of the vertebral bodies. The term spondylosis usually refers to a different stage of the same condition.

Spondylolisthesis
This term is used in the case of anterior or posterior sliding of one vertebral body over another. In some cases the stress placed on the vertebral body can cause it to fracture.

• Ligament injuries
Ligament tissue has only a slight degree of elasticity as its main function is to provide support. If the movement of the spine takes one of the numerous ligaments of the spine beyond its individual elastic limit, it could result in damage to the ligament. Tears of the ligament are known as *sprains*, whereas the term *rupture* is used to describe a ligament that has completely snapped.

• Disc injuries
The term *disc lesion* refers to an injury of the intervertebral discs. The most common is disc protrusion, where the inner part of the disc (nucleus pulposis) pushes through the outer part of the disc (annulus fibrosis), which can in turn make contact with nerves and cause pain (see also nerve injuries).

NEED TO KNOW
In certain cases of overweight and obesity, centre of gravity can be displaced due to the large amount of adipose tissue, which in turn can lead to stress on structures such as ligament and tendon causing postural deviation.

• Muscle and tendon injuries
Many muscles attach to the spinal column via tendons. Both muscle and tendon tissue can only withstand a certain amount of force, after which injury can occur. As with ligaments, tears in muscles or tendons are known as strains, whereas the term rupture is used for a muscle or tendon that has completely snapped.

• Nerve injuries
Nerves that protrude from the spinal column are sometimes disturbed by other structures, such as a protrusion from the intervertebral disc, a narrowing of the spinal foramen or just a muscular spasm. Whatever the cause, any disturbance of a nerve will cause pain. This pain can either be localised or radiate away from the cause of the disturbance. The pain is sometimes given a name that relates to the origin of the nerve that is disturbed; for example, sciatic pain radiates down the leg through the sciatic nerves.

TASK
List the common spinal injuries and give a brief description of each.

EXAMPLE QUESTIONS

1.1 The ulna bone is an example of which type of bone?

    a) long bone

    b) short bone

    c) flat bone

    d) irregular bone

1.2 The patella is an example of which type of bone?

    a) long bone

    b) short bone

    c) flat bone

    d) sesamoid bone

1.3 The pelvis is an example of which type of bone?

    a) long bone

    b) short bone

    c) flat bone

    d) sesamoid bone

1.4 What is the name for the area near the end of a long bone where growth occurs?

    a) diaphysis

    b) epiphysis

    c) periosteum

    d) cancellous

1.5 Which two regions of the spine are secondary curves?

    a) cervical and thoracic

    b) thoracic and lumbar

    c) lumbar and cervical

    d) thoracic and sacrum

1.6 In which region of the spine are the bones fused?

    a) cervical

    b) thoracic

    c) lumbar

    d) sacrum

1.7 Tendons attach to a layer of tissue covering a bone. What is this covering called?

    a) osteoclast

    b) diaphysis

    c) epiphyseal plate

    d) periosteum

1.8 Cells in the bone that are responsible for bone-building are called what?

    a) cancellous cells

    b) osteoblast cells

    c) osteoclast cells

    d) ossification cells

1.9 Cells in the bone that are responsible for breaking down bone are called what?

    a) cancellous cells

    b) osteoblast cells

    c) osteoclast cells

    d) ossification cells

1.10 In terms of postural deviation, an excessive primary curve of the thoracic region of the spine is usually referred to by what name?

    a) lordosis

    b) scoliosis

    c) flat back

    d) kyphosis

1.11 In terms of postural deviation, an excessive secondary curve of the lumbar region of the spine is usually referred to by what name?

    a) lordosis

    b) scoliosis

    c) flat back

    d) kyphosis

1.12 In terms of postural deviation, twisting of the spine is usually referred to by what name?

    a) lordosis

    b) scoliosis

    c) flat back

    d) kyphosis

Further reading

Abrahams, P., Craven, J. and Lumley, J. (2011) *Illustrated Clinical Anatomy* (2nd ed.), Hodder Arnold

Baechle, R.T. (2016) *Essentials of Strength Training and Conditioning* (4th ed.), Human Kinetics

Department of Health (2004) *At least 5 a week: Evidence on the impact of physical activity and its relationship to health.* London: Department of Health

Norkin, C.C. and White, D.J. (2009) *Measurement of Joint Motion: A guide to goniometry* (4th ed.), F.A. Davis

Porter, S. (2008) *The Anatomy Workbook* (2nd ed.), Butterworth Heinemann

Ross, J.S. and Wilson, J.W. (2018) *Anatomy and Physiology in Health and Illness* (13th ed.), Churchill Livingstone

Sewell, D., Watkins, P. and Griffin, M. (2012) *Sport and Exercise Science: An Introduction* (2nd ed.), Hodder Arnold

Tortora, G.J. and Grabowski, S.R. (2017) *Principles of Anatomy and Physiology* (15th ed.), Wiley

Kenney, L., Wilmore, J.H. and Costhill, D.L. (2019) *Physiology of Sport and Exercise* (7th ed.), Human Kinetics

Joints

OBJECTIVES

After completing this chapter, you will be able to:

1 List the different classifications of joints and give examples of each.

2 Distinguish between different types of joints by relating to their range of movement.

3 List and give examples of the different types of synovial joints.

4 Identify the common movements within each type of synovial joint.

5 Identify the typical structures within a synovial joint.

6 List the short- and long-term effects on joints.

7 List the effects of pregnancy on joint stability.

Introduction

This chapter deals with the anatomical system of the body, in particular the classification of joints within the skeletal system from a perspective of structure, function and the effects of exercise. Within the Professional Standards framework, instructors should be able to list the classifications of joints and describe the common structures in each type of joint, as well as describe how exercise can affect joints.

Later chapters provide physiological and biomechanical principles that, together with the anatomical knowledge covered in this chapter, provide the instructor with the understanding and ability to design appropriate exercise programmes for apparently healthy individuals and to understand the effects of various types of exercise on the human body.

Basic types of joint

A simple definition of a joint is the articulation or place where two or more bones meet. In other words, a joint is the place where bones come together. Joints are normally classified according to their structure and function, and there are three broad types: *fibrous*, *cartilaginous* and *synovial*. Fibrous and cartilaginous joints contain connective tissue that binds bone together, whereas synovial joints have a fluid-filled capsule, but no connective tissue binding the joint. Joints can also be classified according to their degree of movement: they can be *non-movable*, such as the plates of the skull which are fused together; *slightly movable*, such as the vertebrae of the spine; or *freely movable*, such as the hip or shoulder.

JOINT CLASSIFICATION

- **Fibrous joints** Fibrous joints, sometimes referred to as fixed joints, are made up of immovable interlocking bones that are connected by tissue fibres. These fibres are mainly made up of collagen, a common tissue in the human body. A joint with bones that are able to move in some way is called an *articulated* joint, therefore a fibrous or fibro joint is a *non-articulating* joint. An example of this type of joint is the skull.

  Fibrous joints need to be very strong to prevent movement of any sort, such as in the joint between the pelvis and the sacrum of the spine. This type of joint is also known as a *suture*. As there is no movement and a high degree of stability associated with this type of joint, the risk of injury is minimal and usually requires great force to do so. If injury to a fibrous joint does occur, however, it is usually extremely painful and slow to heal.

- **Cartilaginous joints** This type of joint has slightly movable bones surrounded by ligaments that strap the joint together, as they do in other joints. Between the ends of the bones that form the joint are pads of *cartilage*, which can be compressed to allow a small degree of movement. Cartilaginous joints therefore allow a certain amount of movement, but also provide a degree of stability. The vertebral bodies and pubis symphysis (pubic bone) are examples of cartilaginous joints. As there is a certain amount of movement associated with this type of joint, the risk of injury is increased. Injury normally occurs with the cartilage discs or articular cartilage, which in most cases does not heal.

- **Synovial joints** Synovial joints are also referred to as freely movable joints as they allow a great deal of movement, with the ligament straps providing most of the support. Unlike the other types, these joints contain a synovial cavity between the articulating bones that allows the range of movement mentioned above. Synovial

joints also have a synovial membrane, which can secrete synovial fluid between the bones in the joint to lubricate the articulating surfaces and prevent friction. Freely movable joints are more susceptible to injury, in particular to structures such as ligaments. Some joints are more stable than others. For example, the hip joint has a deeper ball and socket so is therefore more stable than the shoulder joint, which has a shallower ball and socket. For this reason the shoulder is more susceptible to injury.

TASK
List the three classifications of joint and briefly describe each one in relation to its structure.

TYPES OF SYNOVIAL JOINT

There are several types of synovial joint in the body, and they are classified according to their movement or shape. The types of synovial joint in the human body are as follows (see also chapter 3: The Muscular System for information on the movements):

- **Ball and socket joints** As the name suggests, this type of joint consists of a ball-like end of one bone coming together with a cup-like end of another bone (see Fig. 2.1), for example, in the shoulder and hip joint. A large degree of movement in all three planes is available in this type of joint: flexion, extension, abduction, adduction, rotation, pronation, supination, inversion, eversion and circumduction.

- **Hinge** In this type of joint, the convex end of one bone fits into the concave end of another bone (see Fig. 2.2). As the name suggests, the joint has a motion similar to the hinge on a door (essentially opening and closing) and examples include the elbow, knee and ankle. Only flexion and extension in one plane of movement about a single axis is possible in a joint of this kind.

FIG. 2.1

Ball and socket joint

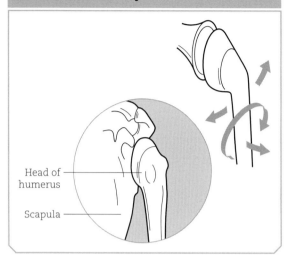

Head of humerus

Scapula

• **Gliding or plane joint** The articulating surfaces of these particular joints are usually flat or slightly curved – for example, the joints made by the carpal and tarsal bones – and the two surfaces glide over each other (see Fig. 2.3). The main movements of gliding joints are side to side and backwards and forwards.

• **Pivot joint** In this particular joint, there is usually a rounded or pointed surface of a bone that articulates with a ring-like surface of another bone – for example, the radioulnar and cervical spine (see Fig. 2.4). The movement is rotational in one axis only.

NEED TO KNOW
The term *synovial* means 'egg-like', as synovial fluid resembles uncooked egg white.

FIG. 2.2

Hinge joint

Humerus

Ulna

FIG. 2.3

Gliding or plane joint

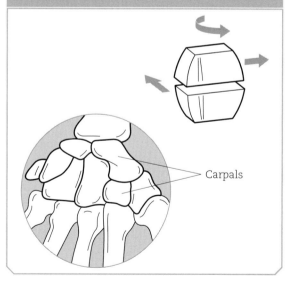

Carpals

FIG. 2.4

Pivot joint

Radius
Ulna

FIG. 2.5

Saddle and condyloid joint

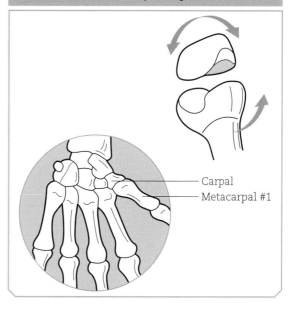

Carpal
Metacarpal #1

• **Saddle and condyloid joint** In saddle and condyloid joints such as the thumb, concave and convex surfaces similar to a rider in a saddle fit together to allow movement in two axes, such as side to side and up and down (see Fig. 2.5). Movements include flexion, extension, abduction, adduction and circumduction.

TYPICAL STRUCTURE OF A SYNOVIAL JOINT

All synovial joints in the body have particular characteristics in common (see Fig. 2.6):

• **Hyaline or articular cartilage** This covers the ends of the bones that form the joint, providing smooth moving surfaces to prevent friction.

• **Capsular ligaments** These 'strap-like' collagen fibres hold bones together to provide support, but also to allow wanted movement.

FIG. 2.6

A typical synovial joint

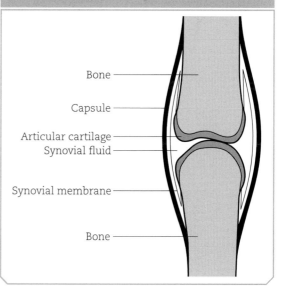

Bone
Capsule
Articular cartilage
Synovial fluid
Synovial membrane
Bone

• **Synovial membrane** This secretes synovial fluid, which lubricates the articular cartilage in the joint.

• **Joint capsule** The joint capsule consists of two layers to provide stability to the joint. The outer layer is a tough fibrous material made up of collagen and elastic fibres and is continuous with the periosteum of the articulating bones. The inner layer is the synovial membrane, which is described above.

• **Synovial fluid** As well as lubricating the joint surfaces, the synovial fluid contains white blood cells, which remove cellular debris, and nutrients, which nourish the articular cartilage. The synovial fluid becomes less viscous (thick) during activity, so mobilisation of the joints prior to intense activity is important.

• **Proprioceptors** There are many receptors in the cartilage and ligaments that provide information to the central nervous system regarding position and alignment.

TASK
List and describe the typical structures within a synovial joint.

TYPICAL JOINT RANGES OF MOTION

Joint range of motion (ROM) is otherwise referred to as joint mobility, which can be affected by many factors such as joint surfaces, muscles, ligaments, temperature, age and gender. The ROM at a specific joint is also dependent on the functional requirement of the individual. In the majority of individuals, a range of motion within normal guidelines is considered suitable. In many cases where the flexibility of an individual joint is considered to be beyond the normal range of motion (often referred to as hyper-flexibility) joint

stability is often lacking or reduced, which can result in a variety of conditions of joint injury. In cases where the flexibility of an individual joint is considered to be less than the normal range, injury such as muscle strain can occur. One of the most accurate methods of measuring joint range of motion is by a technique known as *goniometry* in which either electrical or manual goniometer devices are used to measure individual joint angles. This type of testing is normally carried out by clinically trained and experienced individuals with a view to analysis of restricted movement for those with lifestyle issues or for athletes with specific sport or event requirements. Table 2.1 provides a general overview from a range of published sources of the typical range of motion values (measured in degrees) that are related to specific joints in the body. The lower value in the range represents the point below which possible impairment to the joint is indicated.

The effects of exercise on joints

SHORT-TERM EFFECTS

During exercise, the synovial membrane secretes synovial fluid into the joint in order to lubricate the bony surfaces and thus prevent friction. This is one of the reasons why it is important to carry out mobilisation exercises prior to the main activity, so that the joint can be lubricated before any high-impact or high-intensity exercise is undertaken.

LONG-TERM EFFECTS

Over time, high-impact and high-intensity exercise can damage the hyaline (articular) cartilage that protects the ends of the bones. If this occurs, there may be some damage to the bone itself, resulting

TABLE 2.1

Typical joint ROM values

Joint	Movement pattern	Expected range of movement (degrees)
Shoulder	Flexion	160–170
Shoulder	Extension	40–62
Shoulder	Internal rotation	60–70
Shoulder	External rotation	60–104
Hip	Flexion	90–155
Hip	Extension	9–29
Hip	Internal rotation	26–50
Hip	External rotation	26–70
Hip	Abduction	30–40
Hip	Adduction	10–30
Knee	Flexion	140–145
Knee	Extension	0–5
Ankle	Dorsiflexion	10–20
Ankle	Plantarflexion	30–50

in a condition known as *osteoarthritis*. This can cause inflammation and pain within the joint.

Damage to ligament tissue is common as ligament has only a limited range of elasticity (up to 6 per cent). As blood supply to the ligaments is very poor, the tissues can take a very long time to heal; during the healing process the stability that the ligaments normally provide to the joint can be impaired.

The effects of pregnancy on joints

Due to the influence of the hormone relaxin, which increases in level during pregnancy, connective tissue within ligaments and tendons starts to become more elastic. This in turn will make joints less stable, particularly in the region of the pelvis and lower back. Range of movement will also increase as a result of the joint being less stable. As there is a forward shift in the centre of gravity of a mother-to-be due to the uterus moving up and out of the pelvis, there tends to be an increase in lumbar lordosis (a curved lower back), which can cause considerable back pain. The pubic symphysis (bones in the pubic region) can become less stable and cause pregnancy-related pelvic girdle pain (previously known as symphysis pubis dysfunction), and in some cases separate (known as diastasis symphysis pubis) and can cause severe pelvic girdle pain. In cases such as this, almost any movement of the hips can cause discomfort or pain so it is important to try and minimise this discomfort by keeping the hips aligned and stable. Taking shorter walking strides, avoiding crossing the legs or adduction at the hip, keeping activity low-impact and short duration are all strategies that can help to minimise the pain.

EXAMPLE QUESTIONS

2.1 The tibia and the fibula make what type of joint?
   a) fixed
   b) cartilaginous
   c) synovial
   d) hinge

2.2 The facet joints of the transverse processes of the spine make what type of joint?
   a) cartilaginous
   b) fixed
   c) synovial
   d) hinge

2.3 The tibia and the femur make what type of joint?
   a) fixed
   b) cartilaginous
   c) synovial
   d) fused

2.4 The pubis symphysis is what type of joint?
   a) fixed
   b) cartilaginous
   c) synovial
   d) hinge

2.5 Which of the following is classed as a hinge joint?
   a) shoulder
   b) hip
   c) elbow
   d) wrist

2.6 Which two movements are available at a saddle joint?
   a) pronation and supination
   b) flexion, extension, adduction and abduction
   c) adduction and abduction only
   d) inversion and eversion

2.7 Which of the following make a joint?

a) femur and radius

b) ulna and tibia

c) femur and pelvis

d) phalanges and carpals

2.8 Which of the following make a joint?

a) femur and ulna

b) humerus and scapula

c) sacrum and cervical

d) phalanges and tarsals

2.9 Which of the following make a joint?

a) metacarpals and phalanges

b) fibula and radius

c) coccyx and cervical

d) ulna and tarsals

2.10 Which of the following make a joint?

a) tarsals and tibia

b) pelvis and radius

c) sacrum and thoracic

d) carpals and tarsals

2.11 Which of the following make a gliding joint?

a) bones of the spine

b) bones of the phalanges

c) bones of the carpals

d) bones of the tarsals

2.12 Which of the following make a pivot joint?

a) tibia and fibula

b) atlas and axis

c) cervical and thoracic

d) carpals and tarsals

Further reading

Abrahams, P., Craven, J. and Lumley, J. (2011) *Illustrated Clinical Anatomy* (2nd ed.), Hodder Arnold

Baechle, R.T. (2016) *Essentials of Strength Training and Conditioning* (4th ed.), Human Kinetics

Hamilton, N., Weimar, W. and Luttgens, K. (2015) *Kinesiology: Scientific basis of human motion* (12th ed.), McGraw-Hill

Norkin, C.C. and White, D.J. (2009) *Measurement of Joint Motion: A guide to goniometry* (4th ed.), F.A. Davis

Porter, S. (2008) *The Anatomy Workbook* (2nd ed.), Butterworth Heinemann

Ross, J.S. and Wilson, J.W. (2018) *Anatomy and Physiology in Health and Illness* (13th ed.), Churchill Livingstone

Sewell, D., Watkins, P. and Griffin, M. (2012) *Sport and Exercise Science: An Introduction* (2nd ed.), Hodder Arnold

Tortora, G.J. and Grabowski, S.R. (2017) *Principles of Anatomy and Physiology* (15th ed.), Wiley

Wolfe, L. and Weissgerber, T. (2003) 'Clinical physiology of exercise in pregnancy: a literature review', *Canadian Journal of Obstetrics and Gynecology*, 25(6): 451–453

The Muscular System

3

OBJECTIVES

After completing this chapter, you will be able to:

1 Describe the differences between the three types of muscle.

2 Describe the construction of skeletal muscle.

3 Explain the process of muscle contraction and the sliding filament theory.

4 Distinguish between the properties of fast- and slow-twitch muscle fibres.

5 List and explain the types of muscle contraction.

6 Locate the major muscle groups in the body.

7 List and describe the movements available within the body.

8 Explain the different roles of muscle in the body.

9 Explain what is meant by agonist–antagonist muscle pairing.

10 List and explain the planes of movement of the body.

11 List the short- and long-term effects of exercise on muscle.

Introduction

This chapter deals with the muscular system of the body, in particular the skeletal muscle system, from a perspective of structure, function and the effects of exercise. Within the Professional Standards framework, instructors should be able to list the three types of muscle tissue in the human body and describe the way in which skeletal muscle contracts.

Later chapters provide physiological and biomechanical principles that, together with the anatomical knowledge covered in this chapter, provide the instructor with the understanding and ability to design appropriate exercise programmes for apparently healthy individuals and to understand the effects of various types of exercise on the human body.

Types of muscle

There are three types of muscle tissue in the body: cardiac, smooth and skeletal.

CARDIAC MUSCLE (MYOCARDIUM)

The word *cardiac* refers to the heart; therefore, only the heart contains cardiac muscle. The cardiac muscle contains protein filaments called *actin* and *myosin* (see pages 37 and 38), as does skeletal muscle tissue, but the fibres in cardiac muscle are shorter than those in skeletal muscle. The actin and myosin protein filaments in the myocardium are arranged in disc-shaped cells that allow electrical signals to pass between the cells in order to make the heart contract.

The cardiac muscle is described as *involuntary* as no conscious thought is needed to make it contract. Contraction is initiated subconsciously by the *sinoatrial node* (SA node), which is located in the right atrium of the heart. The SA node automatically generates its own impulses that cause an electrical stimulus to spread across the heart via a network of specialist fibres. This then stimulates the ventricles to contract and pump blood into the arteries (see chapter 7). The SA node is often known as the 'pacemaker'.

NEED TO KNOW
Pacemakers are electrical devices that are fitted to the heart to make it beat when the SA node does not function correctly. Pacemakers can automatically speed up the heart during exercise.

Due to the large number of *mitochondria* (organelles in the cardiac muscle, which use oxygen to produce energy; see chapter 6), the myocardial cells can only contract aerobically. The cells contain large numbers of *myoglobin* (which carries oxygen) and are red in colour. The myocardium extracts a large percentage of oxygen from the blood compared to skeletal muscle. As a result, during exercise the heart has to pump more blood to supply the increased demand.

The blood flow to the heart can be reduced due to a number of reasons – for example, blockages in the blood vessels. A reduced flow of blood to the heart – known as *myocardial*

ischaemia (*ische* meaning to obstruct and *emia* meaning in the blood) – leads to reduced oxygen delivery (*hypoxia*), from which the cardiac muscle cells can die. Individuals who suffer from reduced blood flow to the heart sometimes experience severe pain in the chest, neck or left arm in a condition known as *angina pectoris*, which translates as 'strangled chest'. Hypoxia can eventually lead to a heart attack (known as a *myocardial infarction* or MI) and even death. If an individual suffers from any condition that limits blood supply (*atherosclerosis*), it follows that high-intensity exercise could potentially create a problem for that individual.

NEED TO KNOW
Once cardiac muscle tissue has died it cannot be regenerated by the body. Therefore, the heart becomes weaker.

SMOOTH MUSCLE

Found in the walls of hollow internal structures such as the digestive system, smooth muscle automatically controls the movement of the internal systems of the body. As with other muscle tissue, smooth muscle contains actin and myosin protein filaments, but these are not as regular as they are in skeletal muscle. Smooth muscle also contracts more slowly than skeletal muscle and it maintains its contraction for longer periods. The proteins in smooth muscle are also more elastic than other muscle types.

When smooth muscle contracts, it can cause narrowing of the structures it surrounds. These include the digestive, circulatory, urinary and reproductive systems. Like cardiac muscle, smooth muscle is described as involuntary as its action is controlled by the autonomic nervous system (without conscious thought). For more on the nervous system, see chapter 5.

NEED TO KNOW
Unlike skeletal and cardiac muscle, smooth muscle has considerable powers of regeneration.

SKELETAL MUSCLES

Skeletal muscles are normally attached from bone to bone via tendons to provide movement of the body. They are described as *voluntary* as movement is initiated deliberately.

More than 40 per cent of male bodyweight can be made up of skeletal muscle, whereas for females it can be up to 30 per cent. This varies with age. The largest of this type of muscle in the body is the gluteus maximus, which is the main part of the buttock. The strongest is usually considered to be the quadricep group, even though the jaw can create a greater force. The longest is the sartorius, which runs from the iliac spine in the pelvis to the medial aspect of the tibia (top of the shin bone).

Skeletal muscles

Skeletal muscle will be covered in more detail as this will be the focus of most exercise programmes, although cardiac muscle can also become stronger as a result of cardiovascular exercise.

TYPES OF SKELETAL MUSCLE

Skeletal muscles have many different shapes, but they can be broadly categorised into the following shape groups: parallel, pennate and convergent (see Fig. 3.1).

• **Parallel muscles** An example of this type of muscle is the biceps brachii in the arm, where the muscle fibres run parallel to the long axis of the muscle. In other words, the fibres

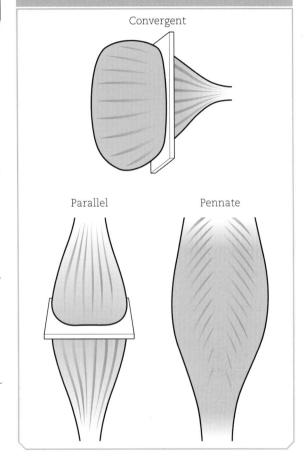

FIG. 3.1

Examples of skeletal muscle shapes

Convergent

Parallel   Pennate

run almost in a straight line from the origin to insertion. Muscles of this type are normally associated with a large range of motion.

• **Pennate muscles** There are two types of pennate muscle: unipennate and bipennate. Both types of muscle have a central tendon for fibre attachment that runs the length of the muscle. In a unipennate muscle the fibres attach to one side of the tendon only, whereas in a bipennate muscle the fibres attach to both sides. The fibres in all pennate muscles attach at an oblique angle and therefore have less range of motion than parallel muscles.

● **Convergent muscles** As the name suggests, convergent muscles have a broad origin of fibre connection that then converges to a narrow insertion. This can be seen in muscles such as the pectorals and deltoids. The range of motion in these muscles is limited, but force generation can be quite high.

TASK
List and describe the basic functions of the three types of muscle tissue within the human body.

STRUCTURE OF SKELETAL MUSCLE

Skeletal muscle is mainly made up of several types of protein. The main proteins that are responsible for contraction are called *actin* and

myosin. Actin proteins are bound together to make thin filaments while myosin proteins are bound together to make thicker filaments. As can be seen in Fig. 3.2, the thick myosin filaments have protruding heads called *cross-bridges*. These cross-bridges 'grab hold' of the actin filaments and pull them in order to cause muscle contraction, using the chemical ATP as energy to do so (see also pages 41 and 90 and 98).

In the muscle, each myosin filament is surrounded by actin filaments. These protein filaments group together to form a *myofibril*, which is the smallest contractile unit (sometimes referred to as a muscle cell) within a muscle fibre. Myofibrils are grouped together to form a muscle fibre. The protein filaments within a myofibril do not run the entire length of the muscle, but are arranged in sections called *sarcomeres*. When the sarcomeres are laid end to end the muscles have a striped or striated appearance. This can be seen in Fig. 3.2: where actin and myosin filaments are in rows, the muscle appears darker, but where the myosin filament has no actin filaments around

FIG. 3.2

Actin and myosin filaments

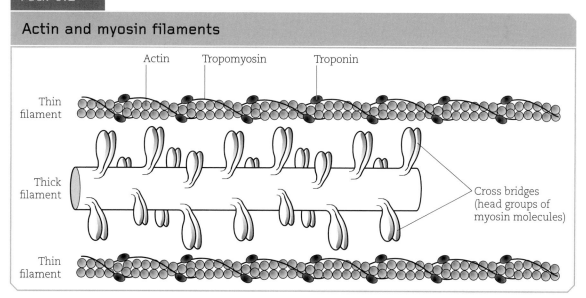

Actin   Tropomyosin   Troponin

Thin filament

Thick filament

Cross bridges (head groups of myosin molecules)

Thin filament

it, the muscle appears lighter. Like all muscles, skeletal muscles have a good blood supply and nerve fibres to pass on the signal to contract (see Muscle contraction, pages 39 and 41).

Each muscle fibre is surrounded by a sheath of fibrous tissue membrane or fascia (meaning bandage) called *endomysium* (*endo* meaning within). This is similar to a sausage wrapped in a skin. The main protein in fascia is called *collagen*. Muscle fibres are then grouped together in a bundle (*fascicle*) and surrounded by another sheath called the *perimysium* (*peri* meaning around). Finally, another sheath called the *epimysium* (*epi* meaning upon) surrounds the entire muscle. At each end of the muscle, the three types of sheath taper off and converge to form an attachment to the bone. These attachment points are called *tendons*. See Fig. 3.3. There are also other structures within the muscle, such as *muscle spindles* and *Golgi tendon organs*, which have specific roles. These two particular types of structure are known as *proprioceptors*, which refers to the way in which information regarding the position of the various body parts is relayed to the brain.

• **Muscle spindles** These specialist cells are sensory receptor cells located deep within the muscles. They relay information to the brain concerning the length of a muscle and the speed at which it stretches. If the muscle in which the spindle is located stretches too fast or too far, the muscle spindle causes a reflex action, making the muscle contract to prevent it becoming damaged. In other words, it causes a built-in safety device known as the *stretch reflex*. The level at which the reflex is initiated is constantly being reset by the brain.

FIG. 3.3

A typical muscle structure

Tendon
Muscle
Epimysium
Endomysium
Muscle fascicles Nucleus
Sarcolemma
Sarcoplasm
Sarcomere
Muscle fibre
Myofibril
Perimysium

It is also important to note that when the muscle in danger of overstretching contracts as a result of the stretch reflex, the opposing muscle (antagonist) allows it to do so by receiving a signal not to contract. This system is called *reciprocal innervation*.

● **Golgi tendon organs (GTO)** These are sensory receptors that lie within the tendon near its junction with a muscle. GTOs are capable of sensing tension in the tendon as a result of muscular contraction or excessive stretching. If this tension exceeds a certain threshold (set by the brain), a reflex operates that causes the muscle responsible for the tension to relax. This is known as the *tendon reflex*.

When skeletal muscles connect to bone, the attachments are known as the *origin* and *insertion*. The origin is the attachment point nearest (proximal) to the midline of the body; the insertion is the attachment point furthest (distal) from the midline. Every muscle has its own nerve supply and is stimulated to contract by the brain sending an electrical impulse or *twitch*. All muscles are in a state of readiness to contract or respond to a signal from the brain. This state of tension has been described as *tone*. By exercising on a regular basis, the amount of muscle tone in the body can be increased, as can the size of a muscle; this is known as *hypertrophy* (*hyper* meaning excessive and *trophy* meaning nourishment). The opposite of this, muscle shrinkage, is known as *atrophy*.

NEED TO KNOW
An example of the stretch reflex is a doctor tapping their patient's knee with a small hammer. The tendon of the quadriceps is tapped, causing the muscle to stretch quickly. The stretch reflex then causes the quadriceps to contract quickly to prevent any danger.

Following a period of strenuous exercise it is common for skeletal muscles to become sore. This soreness, associated with post-exercise self-perception, has been termed *delayed onset muscle soreness* (DOMS). Even though the exact mechanism of this soreness is not fully understood, scientists have found that following periods of intense exercise there is considerable damage at a microscopic level, which may be related to DOMS.

NEED TO KNOW
The gastrocnemius muscle in the lower leg can contain over 1,000,000 fibres.

Muscle contraction

The main function of skeletal muscle is to provide movement for the body through contraction. When a muscle contracts, the protein filaments within the muscle fibre slide over one another with the aid of small projections or cross-bridges. This is known as the *sliding filament theory* (see Fig. 3.7).

Several steps occur before the proteins actually move over each other to cause muscle contraction:

1. The brain sends an electrical signal (or 'action potential') to the muscle fibre via a pathway or nerve known as a *motor neuron* (see Fig. 3.4). The motor neuron has long branches called *axons* down which the electrical signals can travel. A fatty substance called a myelin sheath covers the axon, which helps to conduct the impulse quickly. Each motor neuron can make connections with many muscle fibres, depending on the role of the muscle: in the small muscles of the eye, the motor neuron might make

connection with only a few muscle fibres, whereas in the quadriceps a motor neuron might make contact with thousands of muscle fibres. A motor neuron and the fibres it stimulates to contract are called a *motor unit*. If an action potential is sent, all of the fibres in the motor unit will contract, known as the *all or none* principle. It is not possible to make only some of the fibres fed by the motor unit signal contract.

2. At the end of each motor neuron axon, in close proximity to the muscle fibre to be contracted, is an *axon terminal*. The axon terminal physically spreads out to become larger than the axon itself. This part is called the *synaptic end bulb* because it looks like a bulb and is next to a gap or *synapse*. When the action potential reaches the synaptic end bulb, it causes depolarisation of the covering of the end bulb (the *presynaptic membrane*). Depolarisation is a process in which the movement of sodium and potassium ions (charged particles) causes an electrical current to flow. This is regulated by something known as the *sodium–potassium pump*. The depolarisation process enables a neurotransmitter called *acetylcholine* (Ach), which is stored in the end bulb, to be released across the gap between the presynaptic membrane of the end bulb and the *postsynaptic membrane* (where Ach is collected by the muscle) of the muscle fibre (see Fig. 3.5). The motor neuron axon and the muscle fibres do not physically touch.

3. When enough acetylcholine reaches the postsynaptic membrane of the muscle fibre it can depolarise the membrane. This creates an action potential that stimulates the release of calcium from its store in the *sarcoplasmic reticulum*, which surrounds each myofibril. The calcium uncovers 'binding sites' on the actin molecules that provide a connection for the cross-bridges on the myosin molecules. The cross-bridges are like

FIG. 3.4

A typical motor neuron

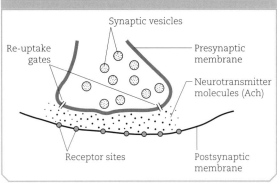

FIG. 3.5

Pre- and postsynaptic membranes

Synaptic vesicles

Re-uptake gates

Presynaptic membrane

Neurotransmitter molecules (Ach)

Receptor sites

Postsynaptic membrane

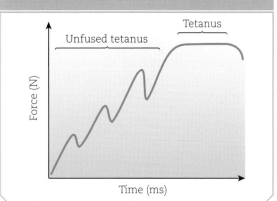

FIG. 3.6

Wave summation and tetanus

Tetanus

Unfused tetanus

Force (N)

Time (ms)

arms that pull the actin and myosin protein molecules across each other (see Fig. 3.7).

4. *Adenosine triphosphate* (ATP) is the fuel within the body that provides the energy for the cross-bridges to pull the actin and myosin proteins (muscle fibres) together. This action is known as muscle contraction.

Each electrical signal (twitch) lasts for a very short time, so the brain needs to keep sending the signals to maintain the muscle contraction. When the brain stops sending the signals, the muscle returns to its original length.

MUSCLE FORCE GENERATION

In order for a muscle to produce and maintain force, twitches need to be sent continuously for as long as the force is required. Also, a single twitch is in most cases insufficient to produce enough force, therefore many twitches have to be 'added' together to produce the required force. This is known as wave summation. Take the example in Fig. 3.6, which shows a required level of force needed for a muscle contraction. It can be seen that the first twitch does not produce enough force, therefore a second and third twitch, etc., is needed to reach the required force. Essentially, after each twitch,

another is sent before the muscular force has time to dissipate thereby increasing the amount of force that was generated by the preceding twitch. In other words, the force is summated each time a twitch is sent. If there is a small amount of relaxation after each twitch, as can be seen in Fig. 3.6, it is known as unfused tetanus. If twitches are sent so quickly that there is no relaxation period it is known as tetanus. In such cases this cannot last for long due to the effects of muscle fatigue.

Types of muscle fibre

Even though there are many different types of muscle fibre, they are usually grouped into two types: fast- and slow-twitch. The term 'twitch' refers to the brief contraction of all the muscle fibres in a motor unit in response to a single electrical impulse from the brain. In slow-twitch fibres each contraction lasts for between 100 and 200 milliseconds, whereas in fast-twitch fibres the contraction lasts for under 100 milliseconds. The two broad categories of fibre differ with respect to the speed and force of the contraction and the type of fuel they use to do this.

FIG. 3.7

The 'sliding filament' theory

Motor neurone

Muscle fibre

(a)

Action potential

Sarcoplasmic reticulum

T tubule

(b)

Troponin

Actin

Tropomyosin

(c)

Active site

Myosin head bound to active site

SLOW-TWITCH (TYPE I) MUSCLE FIBRES

Slow-twitch fibres, otherwise known as slow-oxidative or SO, are the smallest type of fibres and are used for endurance-type activities and posture control. They have many mitochondria (see page 35) and therefore use oxygen and fat as their main fuel source for contraction. The number and size of mitochondria can be increased by endurance training, which means that more oxygen can be delivered to the muscle for the same intensity of exercise, leading to a greater energy output.

Slow-twitch fibres also have many capillaries to supply blood. These fibres are good at

extracting oxygen from the blood as they contain large amounts of myoglobin, which is the oxygen carrier in the muscle. The myoglobin also gives the fibres a reddish colour. As can be seen in Fig. 3.8, slow-twitch fibres contract smoothly and do not generate as much force as fast-twitch fibres, but are more resistant to fatigue.

FAST-TWITCH (TYPE II) MUSCLE FIBRES

Fast-twitch (type II) fibres are powerful, but are quick to fatigue. Generally, they have fewer mitochondria, and therefore use glucose as their

FIG. 3.8

Fast- and slow-twitch muscle fibres

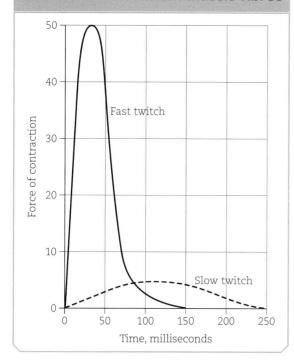

Fast twitch

Slow twitch

Time, milliseconds

main fuel source. As the amount of myoglobin is less, they appear white in colour.

Fast-twitch fibres can be split into two groups: type IIa and type IIb.

● **Type IIa fibres** Type IIa fibres are also known as fast oxidative glycolytic (FOG) fibres because they can use both oxygen (aerobic) and glucose (anaerobic) as a fuel to contract. Like slow-twitch fibres, type IIa fibres contain large amounts of capillaries and myoglobin that allows them to contract aerobically, but also contain stores of glycogen so that they can contract anaerobically. Type IIa fibres can produce more force than type I fibres, but not as much as type IIb fibres. Similarly, the contraction speed and force generation of these fibres is greater than type I fibres but not as

great as type IIb fibres. Type IIa fibres are also known as intermediate fibres because they are between type 1 and IIb fibres in terms of size. Type IIa fibres are used when type I fibres can't cope with the workload of an exercise.

● **Type IIb fibres** Type IIb fibres are also known as fast glycolytic (FG) fibres as they can only use glucose as a fuel to contract. They are the most forceful and largest of the muscle fibres and are used when type I and type IIa fibres can't cope with the workload of an exercise. Type IIb fibres have limited amounts of mitochondria and myoglobin and therefore look white in comparison to slow-twitch fibres. These fibres can generate more force than other types, because the space left due to the lack of mitochondria is filled with more contractile proteins such as actin and myosin. Because the fibres are solely anaerobic, however, they are quick to fatigue compared to slow-twitch fibres.

Table 3.1 shows the common characteristics of the three groups of muscle fibres.

NEED TO KNOW
All muscles in the body contain a mixture of fast- and slow-twitch fibres. This is genetically imprinted from birth.

FIBRE DISTRIBUTION AND MODIFICATION

Most skeletal muscles contain a mixture of all three types of muscle fibre, but their proportion varies depending on the usual action of the muscle. For example, postural muscles have a higher proportion of type I fibres as they are normally required to contract for long periods of time and therefore need to be resistant to fatigue. Muscles such as those of the shoulders and arms, which are not constantly active

TABLE 3.1

Common characteristics of muscle fibre types

	Type I	Type IIa	Type IIb
Contraction time	Slow	Fast	Very fast
Size of motor neuron	Small	Large	Very large
Resistance to fatigue	High	Intermediate	Low
Activity used for	Aerobic	Long-term anaerobic	Short-term anaerobic
Force production	Low	High	Very high
Mitochondrial density	High	High	Low
Capillary density	High	Intermediate	Low
Oxidative capacity	High	High	Low
Glycolytic capacity	Low	High	High
Major storage fuel	Triglycerides	CP, glycogen	CP, glycogen

but are used intermittently to produce large amounts of tension, such as in lifting and throwing, have a higher proportion of type IIa and type IIb fibres.

Even though most skeletal muscles are a mixture of all three types of fibre, the muscle fibres in any one motor unit are all the same. In addition, the different muscle fibres within a muscle may be used in various ways, depending on need. For example, if only a weak contraction is needed in a certain muscle to perform a task, only type I fibres are activated by their motor units in that muscle. If a stronger contraction is needed, the motor units of type IIa fibres are activated in conjunction with those of type I fibres in that muscle. If a maximal contraction is required, all motor units within that muscle are activated. Motor unit recruitment always follows the same order of smaller type I motor units

followed by type IIa then type IIb larger motor units, as can be seen in Fig. 3.9.

FIG. 3.9

Muscle fibre recruitment

Although the number of each type of muscle fibre within a particular muscle never changes, the characteristics of those present can be altered through exercise. Endurance-type exercises, such as running or swimming, result in cardiovascular and respiratory changes that mean the skeletal muscles receive better supplies of oxygen and carbohydrates. This causes a gradual adaptation in the characteristics of type IIb fibres into the characteristics of type IIa fibres. The transformed muscle fibres show a slight increase in diameter, mitochondria, blood capillaries and strength. These changes do not contribute to increased muscle mass. On the other hand, exercises that require great strength for short periods of time, such as weightlifting, produce an increase in the size and strength of type IIb fibres. However, we are what we were born with and can influence the characteristics of our muscle fibres only by a small percentage.

TASK
List and describe the common characteristics of the different types of skeletal muscle fibres.

Types of muscle contraction

Muscle contractions are classified according to what happens to the length of the muscle in the contraction.

ISOTONIC CONTRACTIONS

Isotonic contractions occur when a muscle contracts while lifting and lowering a resistance against gravity. This type of contraction can be divided into two types: *concentric* and *eccentric*. A type of contraction known as *isokinetic* (meaning same speed) is normally used only with specialised testing equipment.

• Concentric contractions

A concentric contraction occurs when the muscle doing the work (the *prime mover* or *agonist*) shortens in length when contracting against a resistance. In other words, the ends of the muscle come together – for example, in the lifting stage of a biceps curl when the weight is being lifted upward. When using free weights, the muscle doing the main work is always contracting concentrically when the weight is moving upward, against gravity. This is slightly different with resistance machines (the system of pulleys means that the limb moving the weight may not be moving upward against gravity, but the weights stack will be), but the muscle doing the main work will be working concentrically when the weight stack is moving up.

• Eccentric contractions
An eccentric contraction occurs when the muscle acting as the prime mover gets longer when contracting against a resistance – for example, when the weight is being lowered during a biceps curl. Here, the ends of the muscle are moving away from each other. In fast movements, muscles working eccentrically have a braking effect.

ISOMETRIC CONTRACTIONS

An isometric contraction occurs when there is no change in muscle length when contracting against a resistance – for example, if a weight is lifted and then held still so that the ends of the muscle do not move either together or away from each other. From a programme design point of view, it is important to be aware that isometric contractions can raise blood pressure.

TASK
Briefly describe the terms eccentric, concentric and isometric.

The roles of muscle in the body

The role of an individual muscle can change depending on the type of exercise or activity it is participating in at a specific time. These roles are normally categorised into the following groups: *agonists*, *antagonists*, *synergists* and *stabilisers*. Table 3.2 describes each role.

AGONIST-ANTAGONIST PAIRS

Muscles are said to work in pairs across joints as they can only pull (contract) and not push. Imagine a muscle pair such as the biceps brachii and triceps brachii in the arm. When the biceps contracts with greater force, it decreases the angle of the joint (flexion), while the triceps stretches to allow this movement. In contrast, when the triceps contracts with greater force than the biceps, it increases the angle of the joint (extension) and the biceps stretches to

allow the movement. If both muscles contracted with the same amount of force or tension, the joint angle would not move.

The muscle that contracts with the most force is called the agonist and causes the joint to move. The other muscle of the pair is called the antagonist. The amount of force produced by the antagonist can vary. Take the example of kicking a ball. The quadriceps muscles are the agonist group as they contract to extend the knee joint. The hamstrings are the antagonist group as they try to control the speed of the extension by contracting slightly. This is known as co-contraction. The amount of co-contraction in the antagonist muscle will decrease through practice of the movement.

When strength training, it is important that both agonists and antagonists are trained to create muscle balance. If either the agonist or antagonist is much stronger or less flexible than the other, the joint that is crossed by the two muscles may be pulled out of alignment to create poor posture. For example, if the quadriceps are much stronger than the

TABLE 3.2

Roles of different muscle types

Type I	Description
Agonist	A muscle that is responsible for the main action or movement (also known as the prime mover). For example, the agonist in a shoulder press is the deltoid muscle group.
Antagonist	A muscle that directly opposes the agonist. For example, the antagonist in a shoulder press is the latissimus dorsi.
Fixator	A muscle that stabilises a joint so the other muscles (agonists) are able to move the levers around the joint. For example, the transversus abdominis is a stabiliser for the pelvis.
Synergist	A muscle that helps the agonist to carry out its movement. For example, the triceps is a synergist for the bench press.

hamstrings, they will pull on the point of attachment at the front of the pelvis (the rectus femoris) and tilt the pelvis forward. In turn, this will lead to an increase in the curvature of the lumbar spine, known as hyperlordosis (see page 19). This is the case for muscle pairs at all joints: there are published guidelines as to typical strength ratios between the pairs (for example, Norkin and White, 2009) that should be reflected in any strength training programme.

Planes of movement

Planes are a useful way of describing movements of the body. The term *plane* is used to describe an imaginary flat surface at various angles to the body. Movement of the human body can occur in three planes: *sagittal*, *frontal* and *transverse* (see Fig. 3.10).

SAGITTAL (OR MEDIAN) PLANE

The sagittal or median plane splits the body into left and right sides (but not necessarily equal halves). The movements distinctive to this plane are flexion and extension. Examples of resistance exercises in this plane include biceps curls, leg extensions, front deltoid raises and triceps push downs.

FRONTAL (OR CORONAL) PLANE

The frontal or coronal plane divides the body into front and back sections. The movements distinctive to this plane are abduction and adduction. Examples of resistance exercises in this plane include lateral pull-downs, shoulder press and lateral shoulder raises.

TRANSVERSE (OR HORIZONTAL) PLANE

The transverse or horizontal plane splits the body into upper (superior) and lower (inferior) sections. The movements distinctive to this plane are medial (internal) and lateral (external) rotation. An example of a resistance exercise in this plane is a chest press.

Exercises or movements can place various amounts of stress on joints depending on which plane of movement is used to perform the exercise. For example, the ligaments in the knee joint allow it to move in the sagittal plane, but are stressed in the frontal and transverse planes. For rehabilitation purposes, exercises are often prescribed in relation to the plane of movement for a particular joint.

FIG. 3.10

Planes of movement

Sagital plane

Transverse plane

Frontal plane

TASK
Choose five resistance training exercises. Name the agonist, antagonist, synergists and stabilisers for each exercise and state the plane in which the movement occurs.

Muscle and movement

As a health and fitness instructor it is useful to know the names and locations (including origins and insertions) of the major muscle groups in the body (see Fig. 3.11 (a) and 3.11 (b)) and the movements

FIG. 3.11

(a) Major muscle groups (front view) (b) Major muscle groups (rear view)

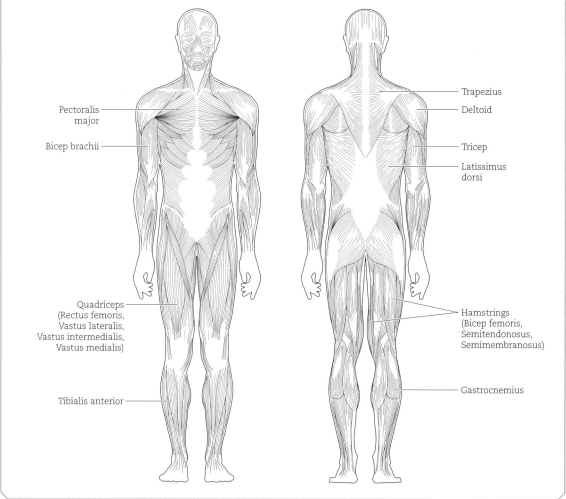

Pectoralis major

Bicep brachii

Quadriceps
(Rectus femoris,
Vastus lateralis,
Vastus intermedialis,
Vastus medialis)

Tibialis anterior

Trapezius

Deltoid

Tricep

Latissimus dorsi

Hamstrings
(Bicep femoris,
Semitendonosus,
Semimembranosus)

Gastrocnemius

FIG. 3.12

Forward flexion of the trunk

FIG. 3.13

Extension of the trunk

they create when contracting. When muscles contract, they either create movement or stabilise the bones that they are attached to. There are many terms used in anatomy to describe movements of the body. It can help to remember some of these movements by linking them to specific resistance training exercises. Common terms and associated exercises are listed on pages 49 and 53.

FLEXION

The term flexion (*flex* meaning to bend) is used when the angle between the moving bones

gets smaller; for example, the forearm coming towards the upper arm in a biceps curl. Another example is illustrated in Fig. 3.12, where the torso is bent forward. This is known as forward flexion of the spine or trunk.

EXTENSION

Extension (*exten* meaning to stretch) is the opposite of flexion and occurs when the joint angle gets larger. An example of this is a straight-leg movement in a backward direction in the sagittal plane, such as a hip extension. Another

FIG. 3.14

Lateral flexion/extension of the trunk

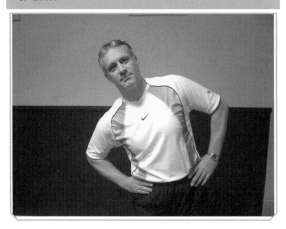

example is shown in Fig. 3.13, where the torso is bent backward from a flexed position. This is known as extension of the spine or trunk.

● **Hyperflexion/extension** The word *hyper* (meaning more than or excessive) in this

FIG. 3.15B

Adduction

sense refers to a movement beyond the normal range of motion for a particular joint.

● **Lateral flexion/extension** This refers to bending to the side. An example is shown in Fig. 3.14, known as lateral flexion or extension of the spine or trunk.

FIG. 3.15A

Abduction

FIG. 3.16A

Rotation

FIG. 3.16B

Rotation

FIG. 3.16B

Rotation

FIG. 3.17A

Medial rotation

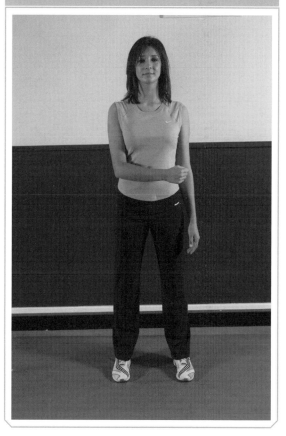

ABDUCTION

Ab means away and *duct* means to lead, and the term abduction is used to describe a movement away from the midline of the body (see Fig. 3.15a). An example is a lateral shoulder raise, where the arm moves away from the body in the frontal plane. Horizontal abduction is a term used to describe the limb moving away from the body in a horizontal motion such as the humerus motion in a seated row.

ADDUCTION

Ad means towards, and the term adduction is used to describe a movement towards the midline of the body (see Fig. 3.15b). An example of this is a lat pull-down. Horizontal adduction is a term used to describe the limb moving towards the body in a horizontal motion such as the humerus motion in a chest press.

ROTATION

This term is used to describe a bone revolving around its own axis – for example, rotation at the ulna–radius joint when turning the palm

face down from a face-up position and vice versa. Another example is the head rotating from side to side, as if saying no (see Figs. 3.16a and b).

• **Medial rotation** This term describes any inward rotational movement – for example, when the upper arm (humerus) rotates towards the body (see Fig. 3.17a). This is a common resistance exercise used for the muscles known as the shoulder 'rotator cuff'.

• **Lateral rotation** This term describes any outward rotational movement – for

FIG. 3.17B

Lateral rotation

FIG. 3.18A

Elevation

example, when the upper arm (humerus) rotates away from the body (see Fig. 3.17b). This is also a rotator cuff exercise.

ELEVATION AND DEPRESSION

Elevation describes an upward movement of a part of the body, such as lifting the shoulders up in a shoulder shrug exercise. Depression refers to a downward movement of a part of the body, such as the shoulders going down from an elevated position. See Figs. 3.18a and b.

RETRACTION AND PROTRACTION

Retraction refers to a movement that involves drawing part of the body back – for example, pulling the shoulders back from a protracted position. Protraction describes a movement that involves part of the body going forward in the transverse plane. For example, when the shoulders go forward, this is known as protraction. See Figs. 3.19a and b.

PRONATION AND SUPINATION

Pronation is used to describe the palm of the hand or the sole of the foot being turned down;

FIG. 3.18B

Depression

FIG. 3.19A

Retraction

supination is used to describe the palm of the hand or the sole of the foot being turned up. See Figs. 3.20a and b.

INVERSION, EVERSION, PLANTAR FLEXION AND DORSIFLEXION

Inversion occurs when the sole of the foot is turned inward, while eversion describes the foot being turned outward. Plantar flexion refers to bending the foot at the ankle joint so the foot is pointing down, while dorsiflexion refers to

bending the foot at the ankle joint so the foot is pointing up. See Figs. 3.21a–d.

Major muscles: their location and available movement

Individual muscles can be responsible for several movements depending on the position of the associated limbs. The following tables

FIG. 3.19B

Protraction

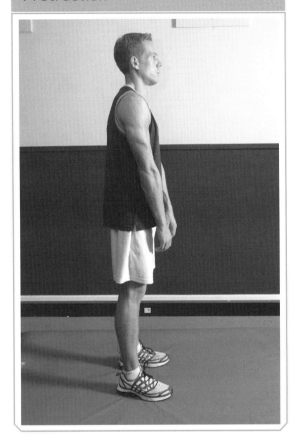

FIG. 3.20A

Pronation

FIG. 3.20B

Supination

provide an overview of the locations and main movements of the major muscles.

TASK

Try to identify all of the major muscles in the body and list their origins, insertions and main movements.

FIG. 3.21

(a) Inversion; (b) Eversion; (c) Plantar flexion; (d) Dorsiflexion

(a)

(b)

(c)

(d)

TABLE 3.3

Locations of the muscles of the shoulder joint/girdle

	Origin	Insertion
Pectoralis major	Clavicle and sternum	Proximal part of humerus
Pectoralis minor	External surfaces of 3rd–5th ribs	Coracoid process of scapula
Serratus anterior	Outer surfaces of upper 8 or 9 ribs	Anterior surface of medial border and inferior angle of scapula
Trapezius	Base of skull (occipital bone) Spinous processes of cervical 7 and all thoracic vertebrae	Lateral third of clavicle Acromion process Spine of scapula
Rhomboid major/ minor	Spinous processes of 7th cervical and upper 5 thoracic vertebrae	Medial border of scapula
Latissimus dorsi	Illiac crest, sacrum, lumbar and lower thoracic vertebrae	Proximal anterior part of humerus
Deltoid	Distal third of clavicle (anterior fibres) and whole ridge of scapula (posterior fibres)	Lateral mid-part of humerus
Biceps brachii (also elbow flexion)	Top of the scapula	Proximal part of radius
Triceps brachii (also elbow extension)	Long head – scapula Lateral head – humerus Medial head – humerus	Olecranon of ulna
Supraspinatus	Groove in top of scapula	Lateral head of humerus
Subscapularis	Underneath of scapula	Medial head of humerus
Infraspinatus	Flat body of scapula	Lateral/posterior head humerus
Teres minor	Lateral medial wing of scapula	Posterior head of humerus
Teres major	Lateral inferior wing of scapula	Medial proximal third of humerus
Levator scapulae	Transverse processes of first 3 or 4 cervical vertebrae	Upper medial border of scapula

TABLE 3.4

Movements of the muscles of the shoulder joint/girdle

	Shoulder flexion	Shoulder extension	Shoulder abduction	Shoulder adduction	Medial rotation	Lateral rotation	Protraction	Retraction	Elevation	Depression
Pectoralis major	x*f*			x	x					
Pectoralis minor							x			x
Serratus anterior							x			
Trapezius								x*m*	x*u*	x*l*
Rhomboid major/minor								x		
Latissimus dorsi		x		x	x					
Deltoid	x*f*	x*p*	x		x*f*	x*p*				
Biceps brachii	x									
Triceps brachii		x								
Supraspinatus			x							
Subscapularis					x					
Infraspinatus				x		x				
Teres minor		x		x		x				
Teres major		x		x*a*	x*a*					
Levator scapulae								x*a*	x	

TABLE 3.5

Locations of the muscles of the hip joint

	Origin	Insertion
Hip flexors: Rectus femoris Iliopsoas (Iliacus/ psoas major)	Bottom front of pelvis Last thoracic and lumbar vertebrae and front of the pelvis	Proximal anterior part of tibia Proximal medial part of femur
Hip extensors: Gluteus maximus	Saccrum, coccyx and medial posterior of pelvis (iliac crest)	Proximal posterior third of femur
Hamstrings: Biceps femoris Semimembranosus Semitendinosus	Ischium for all and biceps femoris has attachment to the femur	Head of the fibula and lateral side of tibia for biceps femoris Proximal lateral posterior part of tibia for other two
Hip adductors: Adductor brevis Adductor longus Adductor magnus Gracilis Pectineus	Pubic bone for all and ischium as well for adductor magnus	Proximal third posterior femur Posterior middle part of femur Whole posterior of femur Proximal inside part of tibia Proximal medial part of femur
Hip abductors: Gluteus medius Gluteus minimus Tensor fascia latae Piriformis Sartorius Tensor fascia latae	Posterior middle part of pelvis for minimus and medius lies above this (ilium) Posterior lateral part of pelvis for TFL. Front of sacrum for piriformis Anterior superior iliac spine for sartorius	Proximal lateral part of femur (greater trochanter) for min and med Proximal lateral side of tibia for TFL Top of greater trochanter for piriformis Upper medial surface of tibia for sartorius

TABLE 3.6

Movements of the muscles of the hip joint

	Hip flexion	Hip extension	Hip abduction	Hip adduction	Hip lateral rotation	Hip medial rotation
Rectus femoris	x					
Iliopsoas	x				x	
Biceps femoris		x				
Semimembranosus		x				
Semitendinosus		x				
Adductor brevis	x			x		x
Adductor longus	x			x		x
Adductor magnus	x*f*	x*p*		x		x
Gracilis				x		x
Pectineus	x			x		
Sartorius	x		x		x	
Gluteus maximus		x			x	
Gluteus medius			x			x
Gluteus minimus			x			x
Tensor fascia latae	x		x			
Piriformis			x*hf*		x	

Effects of exercise on muscle

SHORT-TERM EFFECTS (PHYSIOLOGICAL)

The short-term physiological effects of exercise on muscle include the following:

1. Capillary dilation, which allows for increased blood supply.
2. Increased muscle temperature, which increases pliability (stretch) and power.
3. Increased oxygen demand and usage by muscles being used in order to supply the increased number of fibres being used.
4. The contracting muscle fibres, which squeeze the walls of blood vessels, push blood further

TABLE 3.7

Locations of the muscles of the knee and ankle joints

	Origin	Insertion
Quadriceps: Vastus lateralis Vastus medialis Vastus intermedius Rectus femoris	Whole of femur, lateral, medial and anterior for all vastus (and greater trochanter for lateralis) For rectus femoris see hip joint (page 58)	Proximal anterior part of tibia (via patella into tibial tuberosity)
Hamstrings: Biceps femoris Semitendinosus Semimembranosus	See hip joint (page 58)	See hip joint (page 58)
Calf: Gastrocnemius Soleus	Distal medial and lateral femur (condyles) for gastrocnemius Proximal fibula and medial tibia for soleus	Calcaneus (through Achilles tendon) for both
Tibialis anterior	Proximal lateral half of the tibia	First metatarsal in the foot

along the vessels in a type of pump action known as the 'muscle pump'.

LONG-TERM EFFECTS (PHYSIOLOGICAL)

The long-term physiological effects of exercise on muscle include the following:

1. Improved muscle tone.
2. Improved posture.
3. Increase in muscle bulk (hypertrophy) and strength. This is due to an increase in the number of contractile proteins (actin and myosin), an increase in the number and size of myofibrils per muscle fibre, and increased amounts of connective, tendinous and ligamentous tissues.
4. Increased numbers of enzymes and stored nutrients.
5. Increased number of capillaries and mitochondria in slow-twitch fibres.

NEUROLOGICAL EFFECTS

Strength increases as a result of resistance training can be attributed to neural factors as well as the previously described

TABLE 3.8

Movements of the muscles of the knee and ankle joints

	Knee flexion	Knee extension	Plantarflexion	Dorsiflexion	Inversion
Vastus lateralis		X			
Vastus medialis		X			
Vastus intermedius		X			
Rectus femoris		X			
Biceps femoris	X				
Semitendinosus	X				
Semimembranosus	X				
Gastrocnemius	X		X		
Soleus			X		
Tibialis anterior				X	X

physiological factors. Neural effects include the following:

1. Improved synchronisation in the contraction of motor units.
2. An increased firing rate of motor units.
3. Increased recruitment of additional motor units.
4. Increased activation of synergist muscles.

It is generally understood that strength increases as a result of resistance training are attributed mainly to neural changes in the first few weeks. Hypertrophic changes are usually seen after week five to six as can be seen in Fig. 3.22.

FIG. 3.22

Relative roles of neural and hypertrophic adaptations

TABLE 3.9

Locations of the muscles of the trunk

	Origin	Insertion
Rectus abdominis	Pubis and pubic symphysis	Xiphoid process of sternum and costal cartilage of 5th, 6th, 7th ribs
Erector spinae: (iliocostalis, longissimus, spinalis)	Slips of muscle arising from sacrum, iliac crest, spinous and transverse processes, ribs	Ribs, spinous and transverse processes Occipital bone
Multifidus	Posterior surface of sacrum and processes of vertebrae	Spinous processes 2–4 vertebrae superior of origin
Quadratus lumborum	Iliac crest and iliolumbar ligament	12th rib and transverse processes of upper 4 lumbar vertebrae
Transversus abdominis	Cartilage of lower ribs, inguinal ligament, anterior iliac crest, thoraco-lumbar fascia	Pubis and linea alba
Diaphragm	Xiphoid process Lower six ribs and their cartilage Upper 2 or 3 lumbar vertebrae	All fibres converge to a central tendon
Internal obliques	Iliac crest, inguinal ligament and thoraco-lumbar fascia	Cartilage of last 4 ribs and linea alba
External obliques	Xiphoid process of sternum and costal cartilage of 5th, 6th, 7th ribs	Anterior portion of the iliac crest and linea alba
Pelvic floor: Levator ani and the coccygeus muscles	Inner surface of the pelvis and ischium	Sacrum and coccyx

EXAMPLE QUESTIONS

3.1 What is the main fuel of type I fibres?

a) fat and oxygen

b) protein

c) glucose

d) creatine phosphate

3.2 What is the main fuel of type IIb fibres?

a) fat and oxygen

b) protein

c) glucose

d) alcohol

3.3 Which type of muscle can be found in the digestive system?

a) striated

b) cardiac

c) skeletal

d) smooth

3.4 Which type of muscle can be found in the heart?

a) striated

b) cardiac

c) skeletal

d) smooth

3.5 In muscle contraction, which hormone is released from the end motor plate and crosses the synaptic gap?

a) adenosine triphosphate

b) acetylcholine

c) actin

d) myosin

3.6 Which term is used to describe a muscle under tension where the origin and insertion move away from each other?

a) isometric

b) concentric

c) eccentric

d) isokinetic

3.7 Which term is used to describe a muscle under tension where the origin and insertion move closer together?

a) isometric

b) concentric

c) eccentric

d) isokinetic

3.8 What is the name given to a muscle when performing the role of stabilising a joint?

a) agonist

b) antagonist

c) synergist

d) fixator

3.9 What is the name given to a muscle when performing the role of assisting the agonist muscle?

a) agonist

b) antagonist

c) synergist

d) fixator

3.10 What is the name given to a muscle when performing the main action?

a) agonist

b) antagonist

c) synergist

d) fixator

3.11 Which exercise is associated with the sagittal plane?

a) lateral raise

b) hip abduction

c) pull down

d) leg extension

3.12 Which exercise is associated with the frontal or coronal plane?

a) chest press

b) hip extension

c) pull down

d) leg extension

Further reading

Abrahams, P., Craven, J. and Lumley, J. (2011) *Illustrated Clinical Anatomy* (2nd ed.), Hodder Arnold

Alter, M.J. (2004) *Science of Flexibility* (3rd ed.), Human Kinetics

Baechle, R.T. (2016) *Essentials of Strength Training and Conditioning* (4th ed.), Human Kinetics

Benjamin, H.J. and Glow, K.M. (2003) 'Strength training for children and adolescents', *Physical Sports Medicine*, 31: 19–27

Fry, A.C. (2004) 'The role of resistance exercise intensity on muscle fibre adaptations', *Sports Medicine*, 34: 663–679

Kraemer, W.J. and Ratamess, N.A. (2006) 'Hormonal responses and adaptations to resistance exercise and training', *Sports Medicine*, 35: 339–361

Marieb, E.N. and Hoehn, K. (2019) *Human Anatomy and Physiology* (11th ed.), Pearson

Norkin, C.C. and White, D.J. (2009) *Measurement of Joint Motion: A guide to goniometry* (4th ed.), F.A. Davis

Porter, S. (2008) *The Anatomy Workbook* (2nd ed.), Butterworth Heinemann

Ross, J.S. and Wilson, J.W. (2018) *Anatomy and Physiology in Health and Illness* (13th ed.), Churchill Livingstone

Sewell, D., Watkins, P. and Griffin, M. (2012) *Sport and Exercise Science: An Introduction* (2nd ed.), Hodder Arnold

Tortora, G.J. and Grabowski, S.R. (2017) *Principles of Anatomy and Physiology* (15th ed.), Wiley

4 Cartilage, Ligaments and Tendons

OBJECTIVES

After completing this chapter, you will be able to:

1 Describe the structure and function of cartilage.

2 List and describe the different types of cartilage and give examples of each.

3 Describe the structure and function of ligaments.

4 List and describe the common ligaments found in joints of the body.

5 Describe the structure and function of tendons.

6 List the short- and long-term effects of exercise on cartilage, ligaments and tendons.

Introduction

This chapter deals with connective tissue within the human body, in particular cartilage, ligament and tendon, from a perspective of structure, function and the effects of exercise. Within the Professional Standards framework, instructors should be able to list the types and roles of cartilage and ligament in the human body.

Later chapters provide physiological and biomechanical principles that, together with the anatomical knowledge covered in this chapter, provide the instructor with the understanding and ability to design appropriate exercise programmes for apparently healthy individuals and to understand the effects of various types of exercise on the human body.

Cartilage

STRUCTURE, FUNCTION AND TYPES

Cartilage is a dense, tough connective tissue that forms only a very small portion of the adult skeleton. It consists of a mixture of collagen (*colla* meaning glue) and elastic fibres and has similar properties to plastic, in that it can withstand compression but can tear with combined twisting and compression movements. Cartilage has hardly any blood supply (known as *avascular*), so when it becomes damaged it cannot really repair itself. If it does, the process is slow and not always complete.

There are three types of cartilage in the body: *hyaline* or *articular*, *fibro* and *elastic*. As far as health and fitness instructors are concerned, only articular and fibro cartilage is important as they can both be affected by exercise, while elastic cartilage cannot.

• Hyaline or articular cartilage

Hyaline or articular cartilage is a thin, tough, shiny, smooth bluey-white membrane. It covers the ends of bones that form cartilaginous (slightly movable) and synovial (freely movable) joints, and its function is to prevent friction between the opposing surfaces in joints. This occurs when the cartilage becomes lubricated with synovial fluid, which is secreted by a synovial membrane (see page 25). Moving a joint through its range of movement before an exercise session begins is called mobilisation, and stimulates the release of synovial fluid to prevent friction in the joint during exercise.

• Fibro cartilage

Fibro cartilage is thick, strong and spongy and acts as a shock absorber in joints such as the spine (intervertebral bodies) and the knee (menisci). This type of cartilage is mainly made up of collagen.

• Elastic cartilage

Elastic cartilage is made up of bundles of elastic fibres that provide flexible support. Examples are found in the ear and nose.

Ligaments

STRUCTURE AND FUNCTION

Ligaments are tough, white, non-elastic fibrous tissues strung together in a strap-like formation. They are attached from bone to bone and allow wanted movement while preventing unwanted movement. Ligaments have poor blood supply, so their healing time is slow. Depending on the severity of the

damage to the ligament, it can take weeks to months for the healing process to be complete. However, ligaments can become stronger and in some cases hypertrophy (become larger) following weight-bearing activities.

COMMON LIGAMENTS IN THE BODY

Many ligament structures can be found throughout the body, acting as straps or bindings for specific joints. The following provides an overview of the main ligaments and their function in relation to specific movements at the associated joint. Ligaments allow certain movement to take place at the joint, and for the purpose of this book it is assumed that the ligaments prevent all other movements at the joint.

• Ligaments of the knee

The *medial* and *lateral collateral* ligaments are located on

FIG. 4.1

Common ligaments of the knee

- Femur
- Anterior cruciate ligament (ACL)
- Posterior cruciate ligament (PCL)
- Lateral collateral
- Medial collateral
- Lateral meniscus
- Medial meniscus
- Anterior ligament of head of fibula
- Fibula
- Tibia

the medial and lateral aspects of the knee joint, and allow knee flexion and extension while preventing any other movement. The *anterior* and *posterior cruciate* ligaments are located within the knee joint between the femur and tibia and prevent the two bones from sliding away from each other. See Fig. 4.1.

- **Ligaments of the shoulder** The main ligaments in the shoulder joint are the:

- Coracohumeral ligament
- Glenohumeral (superior, middle and inferior) ligaments
- Coracoacromial ligament

As the shoulder joint is a freely movable synovial joint, it requires a certain degree of movement in all directions. The ligament structures in the joint allow this movement,

but provide stability at the end ranges and prevent the humerus from pulling out of the glenoid cavity (known as a luxation). See Fig. 4.2.

- **Ligaments of the ankle** The ligaments of the ankle can be separated into medial and lateral groups, and the names of the ligaments are taken from the bones to which they attach so they can easily be identified.

The *medial ligaments* are a group of ligaments called the *deltoids*, which comprise the following:

- Calcaneotibial – between the calcaneous and the tibia
- Anterior and posterior talotibial – between the talus and the tibia
- Tibionavicular – between the tibia and the navicular

FIG. 4.2

Common ligaments of the shoulder

Coracoacromial ligament
Coracoclavicular ligament
Coracohumeral ligament
Clavicle
Biceps brachii tendon
Scapula
Humerus
Glenohumeral ligament

FIG. 4.3

Common ligaments of the ankle

Medial view
Anterior talotibial
Tibionavicular
Posterior talotibial
Calcaneotibial
Lateral view
Anterior talofibular
Posterior talofibular
Calcaneofibular

The *lateral* ligaments, known as the *lateral collateral* ligaments, are made up of the following:

- Calcaneofibular – between the calcaneus and the fibula
- Anterior and posterior talofibular – between the talus and the fibula

Between them, the deltoid and lateral collateral ligaments allow the foot to move in flexion and extension, but provide stability in lateral movements such as inversion and eversion. In other words, they prevent the ankle from rolling in or out. See Fig. 4.3.

• Ligaments of the pelvis The
ligaments of the pelvis are required to support a fibrous joint and therefore need to be as strong as possible to prevent any movement whatsoever. The main ligaments of the pelvic girdle are:

- Sacroiliac – between the sacrum and ilium
- Sacrosciatic – between the iliac crest and ischium

There are no muscle attachments across the sacroiliac or pubic joints and so they are dependent on ligaments for stability. Cartilage lines the surfaces of the joints and a pad of cartilage between the pubic bones, at the symphysis pubis, acts as support, shock absorption and to maintain stability and alignment of the pelvis. See Fig. 4.4.

• Ligaments of the hip The main
ligaments of the hip are:

- Ischiofemoral – between the ischium and the femur
- Iliofemoral – between the ilium and the femur

FIG. 4.4

Common ligaments of the pelvis

Ligaments of the pelvis viewed from behind.

Transverse process

Greater sciatic notch

Fifth lumbar vertebra

Posterior sacroiliac ligaments

Greater sacrosciatic ligament

Ischiofemoral ligament

- Pubofemoral – between the pubis and the femur

As the hip joint is classed as a freely movable synovial joint, it requires a certain degree of movement in all directions. The ligament structures in the hip joint allow this degree of movement but also provide a certain amount of stability at the end ranges and prevent the femur from pulling out of its socket called the acetabulum (this is known as a luxation). See Fig. 4.5.

Tendons

STRUCTURE AND FUNCTION

Tendons are bluish-white, slightly elastic fascia tissues that connect muscles to bone. Tendons are made up of the sheaths that surround the muscle fibres and attach to the periosteum covering on the bone. In some cases the area of connection is relatively small – for example, the biceps brachii tendons, but in other cases the tendon can be spread out in sheets over a wide area, such as the tibialis anterior. The latter type of tendon attachment is called an *aponeurosis*.

When muscles contract they pull from the middle and therefore exert a pulling force on the tendons at each end of the muscle. As the tendons are connected to bone, they will attempt to pull the bones together. If one of the bones remains in a fixed position, the other bone will move towards it and create movement.

Tendons stretch only slightly and not as much as muscle tissue, and prolonged tension on tendon tissue may result in tearing. Tendons are reasonably slow to heal as their blood supply is less than that of muscles. As with ligaments, tendons will become stronger with weight-bearing activity.

In the case of extreme force, it is also possible for the tendon to pull away from the attachment point at the periosteum. This is called an *avulsion*. This can be a partial tear, where there is still some tendon attached, or a complete rupture, where the entire tendon is torn from the periosteum. If a complete rupture occurs, the muscle will have no attachment at one end and will therefore be unable to move the bone it is attached to. This requires surgery, whereas a partial tear can heal in time. Tendons can also become inflamed through repetitive use. This type of injury is known as tendonitis (itis meaning inflammation).

FIG. 4.5

Common ligaments of the hip

Ilium

Iliofemoral ligament

Greater trochanter

Pubofemoral ligament

Ischium

Femur

TASK
Describe the structure and function of cartilage (all types), ligament and tendon tissue.

The effects of exercise on cartilage, ligaments and tendons

SHORT-TERM EFFECTS

During exercise, there will be an increased blood supply to both ligaments and tendons. As a result, heat will be produced, which makes these structures slightly more elastic and less susceptible to injury. Also during exercise, synovial fluid is released from synovial membranes in the joints, which lubricates articular cartilage.

LONG-TERM EFFECTS

Both ligaments and tendons are capable of becoming stronger after a long-term period of regular exercise, in particular resistance training. Ligaments can actually hypertrophy (grow in size) by a small amount. An excessive amount of exercise has been linked to damage of both fibrous and articular cartilage.

EXAMPLE QUESTIONS

4.1 What type of cartilage can be described as a thin, tough, shiny, bluey-white membrane?
   a) fibro
   b) elastic
   c) articular
   d) tendonous

4.2 What type of cartilage can be described as bundles of fibres that provide flexible support?
   a) fibro
   b) elastic
   c) articular
   d) tendonous

4.3 What type of cartilage can be described as a thick, strong and spongy shock-absorber?
   a) fibro
   b) elastic
   c) articular
   d) tendonous

4.4 What is fibro cartilage mainly made up of?
   a) elastin
   b) collagen
   c) tendon
   d) fascia

4.5 Which is a ligament of the knee?
   a) coracohumeral
   b) calcaneotibial
   c) lateral collateral
   d) ischiofemoral

4.6 Which is a ligament of the shoulder?
   a) lateral collateral
   b) calcaneotibial
   c) coracohumeral

d) ischiofemoral

4.7 Which is a ligament of the hip?

a) ischiofemoral

b) calcaneotibial

c) lateral collateral

d) coracohumeral

4.8 Which is a ligament of the ankle?

a) coracohumeral

b) calcaneotibial

c) lateral collateral

d) ischiofemoral

4.9 Which type of tissue connects bone to bone?

a) cartilage

b) tendon

c) ligament

d) muscle

4.10 Which type of tissue connects muscle to bone?

a) cartilage

b) tendon

c) ligament

d) muscle

4.11 What is the name of the fibro cartilage in the knee joint?

a) collateral

b) periosteum

c) intervertebral

d) meniscus

4.12 Which type of tissue does the statement 'allows wanted but prevents unwanted movement' relate to?

a) cartilage

b) tendon

c) ligament

d) muscle

Further reading

Abrahams, P., Craven, J. and Lumley, J. (2011) *Illustrated Clinical Anatomy* (2nd ed.), Hodder Arnold

Baechle, R.T. (2016) *Essentials of Strength Training and Conditioning* (4th ed.), Human Kinetics

Porter, S. (2008) *The Anatomy Workbook* (2nd ed.), Butterworth Heinemann

Ross, J.S. and Wilson, J.W. (2018) *Anatomy and Physiology in Health and Illness* (13th ed.), Churchill Livingstone

Sewell, D., Watkins, P. and Griffin, M. (2012) *Sport and Exercise Science: An Introduction* (2nd ed.), Hodder Arnold

Tortora, G.J. and Grabowski, S.R. (2017) *Principles of Anatomy and Physiology* (15th ed.), Wiley

5 The Nervous and Endocrine Systems

Introduction

This chapter deals with the nervous and endocrine systems within the human body from a perspective of structure, function and the effects of exercise. Within the Professional Standards framework, instructors should be able to explain and describe how both systems work within the human body.

Later chapters provide physiological and biomechanical principles that, together with the anatomical knowledge covered in this chapter, provide the instructor with the understanding and ability to design appropriate exercise programmes for apparently healthy individuals and to understand the effects of various types of exercise on the human body.

Overview of the nervous and endocrine systems

Although the nervous system and the endocrine system are separate, they work in conjunction with each other to monitor and regulate all of the systems within the body, including temperature, blood pressure, blood glucose and blood calcium. When the nervous and the endocrine systems work optimally to keep all of the other systems within limits, the body is said to be in *homeostasis*.

The main difference between the two systems is in the way they operate. The nervous system operates as a network of connecting nerve fibres that rapidly transmit electrical signals, whereas the endocrine system operates more slowly using chemical messengers called *hormones* that are secreted into the bloodstream from groups of cells known as *glands*. It is worth noting that when these hormone messengers are released from nerve endings as opposed to glands, they are known as *neurotransmitters*.

Both the nervous and the endocrine systems work on a 'lock and key' basis: the messengers (neurotransmitters and gland hormones) act as keys, and the places they deliver messages to are called locks (or *receptor cells*). Messages will only be accepted by locks if they are the correct keys: in other words, specific neurotransmitters and hormones can deliver messages only to specific sites. If the specific key is not available, there will be no effect on the lock. Take, for example, beta-blockers (commonly prescribed medication for heart conditions). If beta receptor cells combine with beta keys, the resulting message stimulates an increase in heart rate. In the case of cardiac patients, where limiting the heart rate is a necessity, chemicals that block the beta receptor cells, and thus prevent an increase in heart rate, are prescribed. These are called beta-blockers for obvious reasons.

NEED TO KNOW

It was once thought that nerve damage could never be repaired, but scientists have had recent success with regeneration of nerve tissue.

The nervous system

The nervous system has many functions in the body – for example, being responsible for our perceptions, memories and behaviour, as well as being responsible for muscle contraction.

STRUCTURE OF THE NERVOUS SYSTEM

The nervous system is divided into two parts: the central nervous system (CNS) and the peripheral nervous system (PNS). The CNS is made up of the brain, brainstem and the spinal cord (see Fig. 5.1).

The PNS is the part of the nervous system that consists of the nerves and ganglia outside of the brain and spinal cord. The main function of the PNS is to connect the central nervous system (CNS) to the limbs and organs. Unlike the CNS, the PNS is not protected by the bone of the spine and skull, or by the blood–brain barrier, which leaves it exposed to toxins and

FIG. 5.1

The central nervous system (CNS)

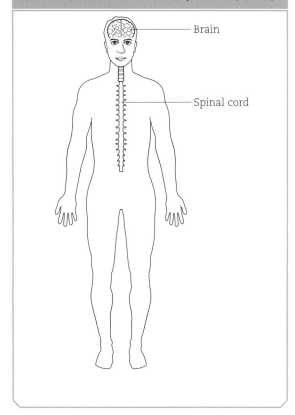

Brain

Spinal cord

mechanical injuries. The PNS is made up of a series of nerve branches that either lead into or away from the CNS. Nerves that lead away from the CNS are called *motor* or *efferent* nerves, as they carry information to muscles and organs to affect a response. Nerves that lead into the CNS are called *sensory* or *afferent* nerves as they carry information back to the CNS about changes in the body.

Nerves that lead into the CNS come from groups of specialised cells around the body called *sensory receptors*. As the name implies, sensory receptors are capable of detecting changes in the body such as temperature, sight, hearing, taste and smell. Table 5.1 lists some receptors and their functions in the body.

TASK

List the common sensory receptors in the human body and give a brief description of what each one does.

When the body is in homeostasis, the sensory receptors do not relay information to the brain. If any changes are detected by the receptors away from homeostasis, information is then relayed to the brain via the sensory or afferent nerves so the brain can initiate a response. For example, if proprioceptors in the ankle ligaments detect that they are being stretched too far, the brain will respond by sending electrical twitches via the motor or

TABLE 5.1

Description of sensory receptors

Receptor	Description
Proprioceptors	These are found in tissue such as muscle, tendon and joints and provide information relating to position. These receptors can be damaged easily in injuries such as ankle sprains. If this occurs, balance can be affected because of a lack of position information being relayed to the brain.
Baroreceptors	This type of receptor is mainly found in the walls of blood vessels in order to relay information to the brain regarding blood pressure.
Chemoreceptors	These receptors monitor the concentration of certain chemicals in the body, such as blood-glucose level.
Thermoreceptors	These are present in all tissues of the body to detect changes in temperature.
Nociceptors	These are present in all tissues of the body and detect pain (tissue damage).

efferent nerves to specific leg muscles in order to balance and stabilise the ankle.

THE CENTRAL NERVOUS SYSTEM (CNS)

The CNS is made up of the brain, brainstem and the spinal cord. All components have different but essential functions and are protected to a certain extent by structures such as the skull and vertebrae.

• **The brain** The human brain is made up of several areas, as can be seen in Fig. 5.2. Each area of the brain is responsible for different functions. For example, the thalamus, hypothalamus and epithalamus are collectively responsible for control of the autonomic actions of the peripheral nervous system. Another example is that of motor skill development, for which the control lies in an area just behind the frontal lobe called the central sulcus.

• **The spinal cord** The spinal cord is a long, thin cord-like bundle of nerve tissue that is covered in a protective layer called the *dura mater*. It extends from the medulla oblongata in the brainstem to the lumbar region of the vertebral column. Its main role is transmission of neural signals between the brain and the rest of the body but it can also function independently by controlling numerous reflexes. To protect the cord from moving too much, the dura mater is tethered at several points along the vertebral column: at the base of the skull, at the sacrum and between each vertebra (see Fig. 5.3).

THE PERIPHERAL NERVOUS SYSTEM

The peripheral nervous system has two branches, known as the *somatic branch* and the *autonomic branch*. The autonomic branch is then further subdivided into two branches, called the

---

FIG. 5.2

The brain and typical functions

Frontal lobe

Thalamus

Hypothalamus: controls body temperature and metabolic rate

Occipital lobe

Cerebellum: receives motor information from motor cortex and peripheral receptors for movement coordination

Spinal cord: links from and to the central nervous system

FIG. 5.3

The spinal cord

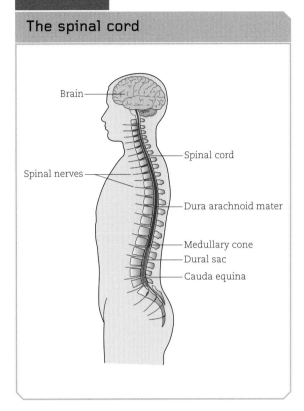

- Brain
- Spinal cord
- Spinal nerves
- Dura arachnoid mater
- Medullary cone
- Dural sac
- Cauda equina

FIG. 5.4

Branches of the peripheral nervous system (PNS)

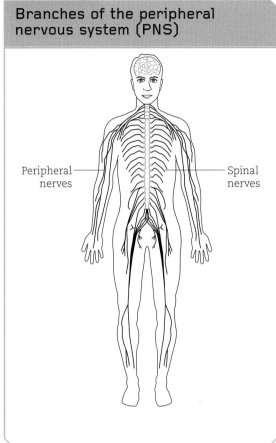

- Peripheral nerves
- Spinal nerves

sympathetic and *parasympathetic branches* (see Figs. 5.5 and 5.6).

- **Somatic nervous system** In simple terms, the somatic nervous system controls voluntary actions such as moving away from danger or foul smells.

- **Autonomic nervous system** The autonomic nervous system controls involuntary actions such as heart rate and blood pressure. This system consists of afferent (sensory) and efferent (motor) nerves. Afferent nerves are responsible for relaying sensation to the central nervous system; efferent nerves are responsible for stimulating muscle contraction. There are 43 segments

of nerves in the human body and with each segment there is a pair of sensory and motor nerves. In the body, 31 segments of nerves are in the spinal cord and 12 are in the brainstem. Besides these, thousands of association nerves are also present in the body. Thus the somatic nervous system consists of three parts:

Spinal nerves: peripheral nerves that carry sensory information into the spinal cord and motor commands.

Cranial nerves: the nerve fibres that carry information into and out of the brainstem. They include the olfactory nerves, ophthalmic nerves, and other nerves that control hearing and balance, facial expressions, and turning of the head and shoulders.

   Association nerves: these integrate sensory input and motor output.

● **Sympathetic nervous system** This branch of the nervous system, also known as the accelerator, acts almost like a stimulus to increase specific activity or stimulate specific processes in the body, as can be seen in Fig. 5.5. Sympathetic nerves do this by releasing the

neurotransmitters *adrenaline* and *noradrenaline* (as discussed on page 84, these are hormones but are called neurotransmitters as they are not secreted from glands). These neurotransmitters speed up processes in the body. For instance, adrenaline stimulates the breakdown of fat and glycogen to be used for energy production.

● **Parasympathetic nervous system** This branch of the nervous system, also known as the brake, has the opposite effect

FIG. 5.5

Sympathetic nervous system

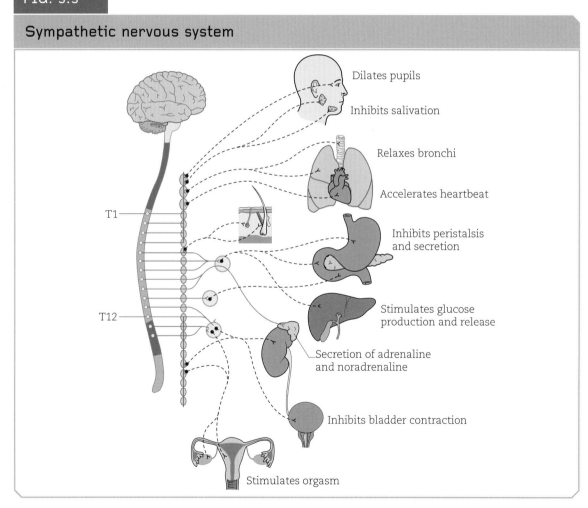

Dilates pupils

Inhibits salivation

Relaxes bronchi

Accelerates heartbeat

Inhibits peristalsis and secretion

Stimulates glucose production and release

Secretion of adrenaline and noradrenaline

Inhibits bladder contraction

Stimulates orgasm

T1

T12

FIG. 5.6

Parasympathetic nervous system

Constricts pupils

Stimulates flow of saliva

Nerve III

Nerve VII

Nerve IX

Nerve X (vagus)

Constricts bronchi

Slows heartbeat

Stimulates peristalsis and secretion

Stimulates bile release

Pelvic splanchnic nerves

Contracts bladder

to that of the sympathetic nervous system: its main roles are reducing the activity of processes within the body and conserving fuel stores, as can be seen in Fig. 5.6. The main neurotransmitter used in this system is acetylcholine (Ach), which is used in the process of muscle contraction (see page 40).

TASK

Draw a diagram of the structure of the PNS, including all the branches.

The endocrine system

As discussed, the nervous system sends messages (information) around the body by using neurotransmitters, which are hormones secreted by nerve endings. The endocrine system is another messenger system for the body that sends messages using hormones (*hormon* meaning to excite) secreted by glands. This is normally done in conjunction with the nervous system: if the homeostasis of the body is disturbed, the nervous system recognises this and in turn stimulates specific glands in the body to release hormones, which try to return the body to homeostasis. Most hormones are circulated via the bloodstream, so the endocrine system can be quite slow compared to the nervous system. As can be seen in Fig. 5.7, endocrine glands secrete hormones. The hormones then diffuse into the blood and are transported around the body. Hormones will only engage with specific receptors; for example, hormones released from the pituitary gland will

FIG. 5.7

Hormone and receptor sites

FIG. 5.8

Glands of the endocrine system

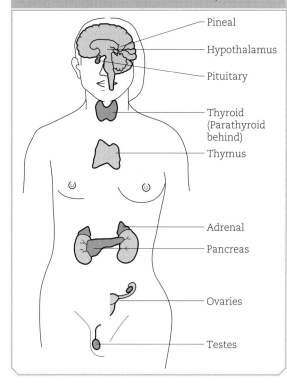

- Pineal
- Hypothalamus
- Pituitary
- Thyroid (Parathyroid behind)
- Thymus
- Adrenal
- Pancreas
- Ovaries
- Testes

NEED TO KNOW
Seasonal Affective Disorder (SAD), which is mainly related to the hormone melatonin, affects about 25 per cent of the UK population.

TYPES OF HORMONES

There are two main groups of hormones: lipid-soluble and water-soluble.

- **Lipid-soluble hormones** One common type of lipid-soluble hormone is *steroid* hormones. Cortisol, testosterone and oestrogen (among others) belong to this group. Steroid hormones take a reasonable amount of time to have an effect, but their effect is usually long-lasting. The main functions of this group are related to either growth function or the control of cycles in the body such as the menstruation cycle.

- **Water-soluble hormones** One common type of water-soluble hormone is *peptide* hormones. Examples include insulin and glucagon, which are used to control blood sugar levels. The main role of this group of hormones is to act on metabolism.

TASK
List the common glands and tissues in the body and the hormones that they secrete.

only bind with specific receptors in the kidneys. Information is then passed on to target cells, which will stimulate the kidneys to perform a specific function.

The main endocrine glands include the pineal, pituitary, thyroid, parathyroid and adrenal glands (see Fig. 5.8). The pineal and pituitary glands are located in the brain, whereas the other glands and tissues are located around the body. There are other tissues in the body that secrete hormones, such as the hypothalamus, pancreas, thymus, ovaries, testes, kidneys and stomach, but these are not referred to as endocrine glands. Table 5.2 provides an overview of the common glands and tissues and their function related to the release of hormone messengers in the body.

HORMONES AND EXERCISE

There are many different hormones in the body and several of them can in some way influence mechanisms related to exercise. Table 5.3 shows a list of hormones considered important to exercise and the physiological functions that they affect.

TABLE 5.2

Roles of the common glands and tissues

Gland/tissue	Role
Pituitary	Produces mainly trophic hormones that stimulate other glands and also growth hormone, which stimulates growth and cell reproduction.
Pineal	Releases melatonin to promote sleep.
Thyroid	Tyrosine-based hormones that regulate metabolism.
Parathyroid	Produces hormones that control bone growth by regulating calcium levels in the body.
Adrenal glands	Produces hormones such as adrenaline, cortisol, aldesterone and noradrenaline (catecholamines and corticosteroids are group names) which are responsible for the increase in nutrient breakdown and also stress response.
Pancreas	Responsible for the production of insulin and glucagon into the bloodstream in order to control blood sugar levels.
Testes and ovaries	Produces sex hormones such as testosterone and oestrogen to regulate reproductive function.

There are many hormonal responses to cardio and resistance exercise in both the short term and the long term. With exercise, there is an immediate increase in hormones such as epinephrine and norepinephrine. These hormones are responsible for increasing blood glucose levels and are important for increasing force production, muscle contraction rate, and energy production (i.e. the synthesis of ATP). It is thought that this rise in hormones begins before the exercise as an anticipatory response to the challenge ahead (Kraemer and Ratamess 2005). Although research as to the effects of exercise is limited, Table 5.4 lists selected hormones and describes their general response to regular exercise.

HORMONES AND OVER-TRAINING

The term 'over-training' is generally considered to relate to a physiological and psychological state brought about by an excessive amount of training over a long period of time. The term 'over-reaching' tends to be used for similar situations but is related to occurrence in the short term. In other words, over-reaching can lead to over-training. Any increase in training volume and/or intensity resulting in long-term performance decrements may result in neuroendocrine changes. Such changes include reduced resting levels of testosterone and insulin-like growth factor (IGF) and significant increases in cortisol levels, which negatively affects the rate of protein synthesis.

TABLE 5.3

Exercise-related hormones and their effects

Hormone	Function
Human growth hormone (HGH)	A peptide hormone secreted by the anterior pituitary gland that stimulates cellular growth. HGH can increase muscle protein synthesis, increase bone mineralisation and promote fat metabolism. It is thought to be stimulated by high-intensity exercise such as heavy strength training, explosive power training or high-intensity cardio exercise.
Insulin-like growth factor (IGF)	IGF is a peptide hormone produced in the liver that supports the function of HGH to repair protein damaged during exercise.
Testosterone	A steroid hormone produced mainly by the testes in males and the ovaries in females. Testosterone is responsible for muscle protein re-synthesis (significant role in skeletal muscle growth).
Insulin	A peptide hormone produced by the pancreas. Insulin regulates carbohydrate and fat metabolism and promotes storage of glucose.
Glucagon	Glucagon is produced by the pancreas. It increases blood glucose levels and stimulates the release of free fatty acids (FFAs) from adipose tissue. As exercise continues, glucagon releases glycogen stored in the liver to provide a source of glucose.
Cortisol	A steroid hormone produced by the adrenal gland in response to exercise (as well as stress). Cortisol is involved in the breakdown of triglyceride and protein to produce glucose. Extended exercise can increase cortisol levels resulting in the breakdown (catobolisation) of protein for fuel.
Epinephrine and norepinephrine	These hormones are classified as catecholamines and are produced by the adrenal glands. Epinephrine elevates cardiac output, increases blood glucose and supports fat metabolism. Norepinephrine performs similar functions as epinephrine and is also involved in vasoconstriction to parts of the body not involved in exercise.
Corticotropin	This hormone stimulates the adrenal glands to increase fat metabolization for energy.

TABLE 5.4

Exercise-related hormones and their training response

Hormone	Training response
Growth hormone (GH)	Most research involves response to single sessions. Resting values are increased but less so in trained people.
Testosterone	Most research involves response to single sessions. Resting values are increased but less so in trained people. Most studies used male subjects. No changes found yet in women.
Cortisol	Cortisol levels increase less in trained than in untrained people.
Epinephrine and norepinephrine	Levels decrease progressively with training. This can result in lower heart rate and blood pressure levels during sub-maximal exercise (lowering the oxygen demand for a given intensity).
Insulin and glucagon	Long-term exercise can result in improved insulin sensitivity.
Follicle-stimulating hormone (FSH) and luteinising hormone (LH)	Regular exercise can depress reproductive hormones such as oestrogen, which may in turn reduce breast cancer risk; however, excessive amounts of exercise may cause menstrual dysfunction.

EXAMPLE QUESTIONS

5.1 Glands are responsible for secreting what into the bloodstream?
a) glucose
b) neurotransmitters
c) hormones
d) ATP

5.2 Nerve endings are responsible for secreting what?
a) neurotransmitters
b) ATP
c) hormones
d) glucose

5.3 Nerves that lead away from the central nervous system are known as what?
a) motor or afferent
b) motor or efferent
c) sensory or efferent
d) sensory or afferent

5.4 Nerves that lead back to the central nervous system are known as what?
a) sensory or afferent
b) sensory or efferent
c) motor or efferent
d) motor or afferent

5.5 Which of the following receptors sense position?
a) proprioceptors
b) chemoreceptors
c) nociceptors
d) thermoreceptors

5.6 Which of the following receptors sense pain?
a) proprioceptors
b) chemoreceptors
c) nociceptors

d) thermoreceptors

5.7 Which of the following receptors sense temperature?

a) proprioceptors

b) chemoreceptors

c) nociceptors

d) thermoreceptors

5.8 Which of the following receptors sense chemical composition?

a) proprioceptors

b) chemoreceptors

c) nociceptors

d) thermoreceptors

5.9 Catecholamines and corticosteroids are secreted by which gland?

a) pituitary

b) parathyroid

c) pancreas

d) adrenals

5.10 Tyrosine-based hormones that regulate metabolism are secreted by which gland?

a) pituitary

b) thyroid

c) pancreas

d) adrenals

5.11 Glucagon is secreted by which gland?

a) pituitary

b) parathyroid

c) pancreas

d) adrenals

5.12 Testosterone and oestrogen are secreted by which gland?

a) pituitary

b) parathyroid

c) pancreas

d) testes and ovaries

Further reading

Abrahams, P., Craven, J. and Lumley, J. (2011) *Illustrated Clinical Anatomy* (2nd ed.), Hodder Arnold

Baechle, R.T. (2016) *Essentials of Strength Training and Conditioning* (4th ed.), Human Kinetics

Kraemer, W.J. and Ratamess, N.A. (2005) 'Hormonal responses and adaptations to exercise and training', *Sports Medicine*, 35(4): 339-361

Porter, S. (2008) *The Anatomy Workbook* (2nd ed.), Butterworth Heinemann

Ross, J.S. and Wilson, J.W. (2018) *Anatomy and Physiology in Health and Illness* (13th ed.), Churchill Livingstone

Sewell, D., Watkins, P. and Griffin, M. (2012) *Sport and Exercise Science: An Introduction* (2nd ed.), Hodder Arnold

Tortora, G.J. and Grabowski, S.R. (2017) *Principles of Anatomy and Physiology* (15th ed.), Wiley

6 Energy Systems

OBJECTIVES

After completing this chapter, you will be able to:

1 Name and describe the structure of ATP used for muscle contraction.
2 Name and describe each system within the body that can produce ATP.
3 Explain how each energy-producing system is contributing at low, medium and high exercise intensities.
4 Name the by-products of each energy-producing system.
5 Explain the problems associated with lactic acid.
6 Suggest ways to prevent depletion of glucose stores in the body.
7 Name typical activities associated with each energy-producing system as the main contributing system.
8 Explain how fitness levels can affect the energy-producing systems being used.
9 Describe the process of excess post-exercise oxygen consumption (EPOC).

Introduction

This chapter deals with the supply of fuel to the muscles of the body, known as *energy systems*, and in particular the interaction of the various systems during rest and during different intensities of exercise. Within the Professional Standards framework, instructors should be able to describe each of the different systems as well as describe how these interact during rest and exercise.

This chapter provides the instructor with the understanding of how energy systems work, which will provide the underpinning knowledge to assist in the design of appropriate exercise programmes for apparently healthy individuals and in understanding the effects of various types of exercise on the human body.

Energy systems for muscular contraction

Whether the body is at rest or moving, energy must be supplied either to living systems for chemical reactions to take place or to the muscles for movement to occur. The unit of energy that is used in the body for muscles to contract is called *adenosine triphosphate* (ATP), which is sometimes known as the *energy currency* in the body.

An ATP molecule is made up of the adenosine part (a molecule of adenine and a molecule of ribose) with three (*tri* meaning three) phosphate groups bonded to each other (see Fig. 6.1).

The bonds keeping the phosphates together are known as *high-energy bonds*. If one of the phosphates is split from the adenosine molecule, a large amount of energy is released to be used for muscle contraction (see Fig. 6.2). Heat is also given off when a phosphate splits from the adenosine. This leaves an adenosine molecule with only two phosphates, which is called *adenosine diphosphate* or ADP (*di* meaning two).

The main problem with this is that there is only enough ATP in the body to last for about four seconds, so a phosphate must be re-attached to the ADP to make ATP in order for the process to start again. This is called *re-synthesis*. Carbohydrates, fats and proteins are digested to provide a source of phosphate.

This process of re-synthesis occurs on a continuous basis in the body, but the amount of energy in the form of ATP that is needed depends on the amount of muscle contraction or exercise being carried out: obviously, when exercising at a higher level, more ATP is needed to supply the energy. The places in the muscle where the ATP is used to provide energy for muscle contraction are called the *mitochondria* (see page 35) or the 'powerhouses'.

Carbohydrates are used to supply energy in the form of ATP mainly in the short term, and

FIG. 6.1

An ATP molecule

FIG. 6.2

Phosphate splitting from an ATP molecule

Adenosine   Phosphate   Phosphate

✷ = Energy release from ATP

fats are used mainly in the long term. Protein is usually used only as a standby source of ATP energy. There are three systems within the body that supply the energy from the digested food to the muscles that need it: the creatine phosphate (ATP–CP) system, the *aerobic* system and the *anaerobic* system.

THE CREATINE PHOSPHATE SYSTEM (ATP–CP)

This system is also known as the PCr or *phosphocreatine* system. As ATP stores last only for a few seconds, the body needs a system that can re-synthesise ADP to ATP very quickly when an individual starts to exercise. The creatine phosphate system can do this almost immediately, but the body contains only a very short-term supply. As a result, the system can be used for up to about 10 seconds only, but can be used over and over again as long as a recovery period of about three minutes is allowed (this recovery period can be low-intensity exercise). Once the creatine phosphate molecule has given its phosphate to the ADP, which in turn becomes ATP, a phosphate can be broken off to release energy (see Fig. 6.3).

This system is very simple and produces no waste products. However, it is not very efficient: for every one molecule of creatine phosphate used, only one molecule of ATP is produced. After the store of creatine phosphate in the body has been used, the body must switch to another system to supply phosphate in order to

FIG. 6.3

The ATP–CP system

Phosphate · Phosphates · Adenosine · Creatine · ✸ = Energy release from ATP

FIG. 6.4

The anaerobic system

Lactic Acid · Glucose · ✸ = Energy release from ATP

re-synthesise ADP. Imagine this system in terms of driving a car. The creatine phosphate system is the first system to be used in the body, just like first gear is the first gear to be used in a car. If you were to drive a long distance in first gear, the amount of fuel used would be enormous and therefore not very efficient. This is the same in the body: if you used only creatine phosphate as an energy source, it would run out very quickly. The body needs to move into another system to provide energy, just like the car needs to move into second gear. However, it must be noted that all energy systems are active at the same time.

THE ANAEROBIC OR LACTIC ACID SYSTEM

● **Glucose (without oxygen)** Glucose is a sugar found in carbohydrate foods such as potatoes, vegetables, rice, bread and fruit. When carbohydrates are digested they release glucose, which is then stored in the body as *glycogen*. Glucose in the blood or glycogen from stores in the body are then used to supply phosphates. The process of breaking down glucose to provide energy is called *anaerobic glycolysis*.

If the exercise intensity is high, this energy supply system can be maintained continuously only for two to three minutes, as it produces a substance called *lactic acid* as a waste product (see Fig. 6.4). Lactic acid can stop muscle contraction if too much is produced, and the

greater the intensity of exercise, the more lactic acid is produced.

As this is the next system that the body uses to supply energy after the ATP–CP system, it is equivalent to using second gear in a car. If you were going on a long journey in a car, you would again use a lot of fuel if you stayed in this gear for the entire journey. It is the same in the body: only two ATP molecules are produced from each glucose molecule, so the body needs to move on to the next, more efficient system or gear.

THE AEROBIC SYSTEM

● **Glucose (with oxygen)** After a few minutes of exercise, oxygen is transported to the muscles to be used with glucose to provide energy in a system called *aerobic glycolysis*. As long as the intensity is not too high, and oxygen is present, there will be no build-up of lactic acid. Carbon dioxide and water are given off as waste products (see Fig. 6.5).

FIG. 6.5

The aerobic system using glucose

Glucose · Oxygen · $CO_2 + H_2O$ · ✸ = Energy release from ATP

When oxygen is used in re-synthesis it is more efficient, as 38 molecules of ATP are produced per molecule of oxygen. However, one of the problems with this system is that there is only sufficient glycogen stored in the body for medium intensity exercise of about two hours duration, if the storage is full prior to the exercise; if glycogen stores have been used up in previous exercise and haven't yet been replaced, the possible duration of exercise using this system will be less. This is similar to going on a long journey in a car and having a less than full fuel tank – either you can't travel as far, or you need to re-fuel. Carbohydrate drinks can be taken during exercise to supply glucose to the muscles; this also spares the stores in the body. It is also important to eat a carbohydrate snack as soon as possible after exercise to replace glucose that has been used during the exercise. However, rather than rely on this system for energy, the body has another system that is even more efficient and uses fat, among other things, as a fuel.

● **Fat (with oxygen)** After several minutes of exercise (this time varies with fitness levels) intramuscular fat or fat that is transported to the muscle can be used in the energy process. In order for this to happen, small amounts of glucose and oxygen must be available. The place in the muscle where energy is released by breaking down fat, carbohydrate and oxygen is called the *mitochondria*. There is no build-up of lactic acid, but carbon dioxide,

water and heat are given off as by-products (see Fig. 6.6). This system is used when the exercise is of low-to-moderate intensity, such as walking or comfortable jogging. As this system uses a small amount of glucose, the exercise can be maintained only as long as glucose is available, usually about two hours (less if the exercise was started on low stores of glucose), unless carbohydrates are taken in during the exercise.

Note: There are other ways to metabolise fat which are beyond the scope of this book.

Depending on the type of fat used in this system (there are several types of fat available from food), more than 200 ATP molecules can be produced from each molecule of fat, glucose and oxygen. This makes this system very efficient in producing energy for muscle contraction. However, if stores of glucose do run out, it can be difficult for the body to break down fat. This is another reason why carbohydrate foods are important when exercising.

A person who exercises on a regular basis will move through the systems, like the gears in a car, to get to the system using fat more quickly than a person who is not used to exercise. This is simply because the body responds to the exercise regularity by becoming more efficient.

Interaction of energy systems

The body actually uses all of the above systems at the same time; however, the intensity of the exercise dictates which energy system will be used to supply the majority of the energy (see Fig. 6.7).

For example, at the start of exercise (warm-up) the demand for oxygen cannot be met quickly by the aerobic system, so the anaerobic system must contribute more to energy production. However, as the warm-up continues

The aerobic system using fat

Fat + Oxygen → $CO_2 + H_2O$ ✸ = Energy release from ATP

FIG. 6.7

Interaction of energy systems

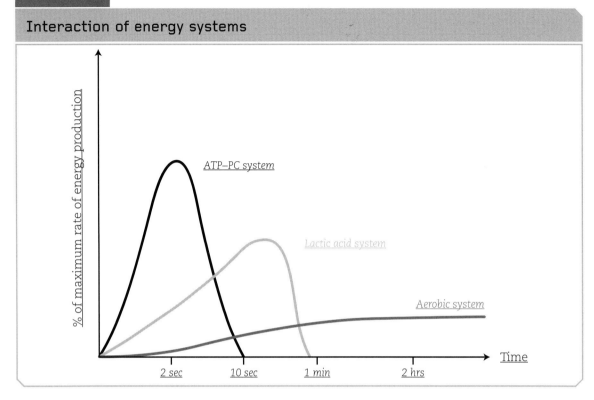

the capillaries in the lungs and muscles dilate, increasing the flow of oxygen so that the contribution from the aerobic systems increases. After a period of time, which in some cases can be up to 30 minutes or more (at low to medium intensity), most of the energy is provided by the fat system, with the other systems providing a small amount. If, during low- to medium-intensity exercise, the individual decides to increase to a high intensity, the sudden requirement for extra energy usually comes from extra glucose in the body.

However, the problem here is that large amounts of glucose will be needed to provide the large amount of energy required to sustain the high-intensity exercise. This means that large amounts of the by-product lactic acid will be produced, which will eventually stop

the muscle from contracting. High-intensity exercise producing large amounts of lactic acid is normally only sustainable for about two minutes, and much less in unfit people.

Table 6.1 shows the main energy systems used in typical sporting activities.

Excess post-exercise oxygen consumption

Sometimes referred to as *afterburn*, excess post-exercise oxygen consumption (EPOC) can be described as 'the amount of oxygen above resting requirements for a period of time

TABLE 6.1

Major energy systems used in typical activities

Major energy system	Performance time	Typical activities
ATP–CP	<10 seconds	Shot-put
		100m sprints
Anaerobic glycolysis	20–90 seconds	200–400m sprints
		Speed skating
		100m swim
Aerobic glycolysis	90 seconds to several minutes	Gymnastics
		800m run
		Boxing round
Fat	More than several minutes	Jogging

after exercise has finished'. It was originally referred to (as far back as 1923 by Hill and Lupton) as the oxygen debt. The term oxygen debt has since been replaced by the more appropriate term excess post-exercise oxygen consumption (EPOC). In simple terms, after a period of exercise the body continues to burn more calories until it returns back to its pre-exercise state. Generally speaking, the more intense the exercise, the greater the amount of calories used due to EPOC, which is why High Intensity Interval Training (HIIT) is regarded as a good strategy for weight loss goals as it has a more pronounced effect on EPOC than aerobic exercise (as does resistance training). It should be emphasised, however, that better effects are related to higher intensity resistance training; therefore, those new to this type of training should undergo a period of familiarisation followed by a progressive programme. It should also be noted that any weight-loss benefits due to resistance training and EPOC would occur over a significant time period; therefore, a combination of cardio and resistance exercises should be promoted.

EXAMPLE QUESTIONS

6.1 When a phosphate molecule is split from ATP what does it leave?

a) creatine

b) CP

c) AMP

d) ADP

6.2 What is the main process that occurs within mitochondria?

a) production of ATP without the presence of oxygen

b) production of ATP in the presence of oxygen

c) converting glucose to glycogen in the presence of oxygen

d) converting glucose to glycogen without the presence of oxygen

6.3 Anaerobic glycolysis is ...

a) breaking down glucose in the presence of oxygen

b) breaking down glucose without the presence of oxygen

c) converting glucose to glycogen in the presence of oxygen

d) converting glucose to glycogen without the presence of oxygen

6.4 Aerobic glycolysis is ...

a) breaking down glucose in the presence of oxygen

b) breaking down glucose without the presence of oxygen

c) converting glucose to glycogen in the presence of oxygen

d) converting glucose to glycogen without the presence of oxygen

6.5 Which of the following is given off as a by-product of aerobic glycolysis?

a) ATP

b) hydrogen

c) lactic acid

d) carbon dioxide and water

6.6 Which of the following is given off as a by-product of anaerobic glycolysis?

a) ATP

b) hydrogen

c) lactic acid

d) carbon dioxide and water

6.7 Which of the following is produced as a result of incomplete breakdown of fat due to lack of available carbohydrate?

a) lactic acid

b) hydrogen

c) ketones

d) carbon dioxide and water

6.8 Which energy system contributes the most (in percentage terms) at the start of exercise?

a) anaerobic glycolysis

b) aerobic glycolysis

c) ATP–PC system

d) fat

6.9 Which energy system contributes the least (in percentage terms) at the start of exercise?

a) anaerobic glycolysis

b) aerobic glycolysis

c) ATP–PC system

d) aerobic (fat)

6.10 Which energy system contributes the most (in percentage terms) in short sprint events such as the 100 metres?

a) anaerobic glycolysis

b) aerobic glycolysis

c) ATP–PC system

d) aerobic (fat)

6.11 Which energy system contributes the most (in percentage terms) in events such as the 800 metres?

a) they are all the same

b) aerobic glycolysis

c) ATP–PC system

d) lactic acid system

6.12 Which energy system contributes the most (in percentage terms) in events such as a long distance run?

a) they are all the same

b) aerobic (fat)

c) ATP–PC system

d) lactic acid system

Further reading

Abrahams, P., Craven, J. and Lumley, J. (2011) *Illustrated Clinical Anatomy* (2nd ed.), Hodder Arnold

Baechle, R.T. (2016) *Essentials of Strength Training and Conditioning* (4th ed.), Human Kinetics

Gastin, P.B. (2001) 'Energy system interaction and relative contribution during maximal exercise', *Sports Medicine*, 31: 725–741

Hargreaves, M. and Spriet, L. (2006) *Exercise Metabolism* (2nd ed), Human Kinetics

Hill, A.V. and Lupton, H. (1923) 'Muscular Exercise, Lactic Acid and the Supply and Utilisation of Oxygen', *Quarterly Journal of Medicine*, 16, 135

McArdle, W.D., Katch, F.I. and Katch, V.L. (2007) *Exercise Physiology* (6th ed.), Lippincott, Williams & Wilkins

Maud, P. and Foster, C. (2006) *Physiological Assessment of Human Fitness* (2nd ed.), Human Kinetics

Mougios, V. (2006) *Exercise Biochemistry*, Human Kinetics

Porter, S. (2008) *The Anatomy Workbook* (2nd ed.), Butterworth Heinemann

Ross, J.S. and Wilson, J.W. (2018) *Anatomy and Physiology in Health and Illness* (13th ed.), Churchill Livingstone

Sewell, D., Watkins, P. and Griffin, M. (2012) *Sport and Exercise Science: An Introduction* (2nd ed.), Hodder Arnold

Tortora, G.J. and Grabowski, S.R. (2017) *Principles of Anatomy and Physiology* (15th ed.), Wiley

7 The Heart and the Circulatory System

OBJECTIVES

After completing this chapter, you will be able to:

1   Describe the structure of the heart in relation to the layers of muscle and surrounding sheath.

2   Name and describe the sections within the heart.

3   Explain the process of heart contraction (cardiac cycle).

4   Describe the flow of blood into and away from the heart and describe the features of the associated vessels.

5   Describe the composition of blood.

6   Explain the mechanisms of venous return.

7   Explain the terms *hypertension* and *hypotension* in relation to blood pressure and how exercise affects blood pressure.

8   Explain the short- and long-term effects of exercise on the heart and circulation system.

9   Describe the key cardiovascular differences in various population groups.

Introduction

This chapter deals with the anatomical system of the body in relation to the cardiac and circulatory systems (known as the cardiovascular system) from the perspective of structure, function and the effects of exercise. Within the Professional Standards framework, instructors should be able to describe the common structures of both systems and describe their functions, as well as describe how exercise can impact on the systems.

Later chapters in the book provide physiological and biomechanical principles that, together with the knowledge of the cardiovascular system covered in this chapter, will provide you with the understanding and ability to design appropriate exercise programmes for apparently healthy individuals and to understand the effects of various types of exercise on the human body.

The cardiopulmonary system

The system that supplies oxygen and nutrients to the muscles and takes away waste products such as carbon dioxide is called the cardiopulmonary system, and is made up of the lungs, heart and associated vessels (see Fig. 7.1). The lungs provide the system that delivers oxygen to and extracts carbon dioxide from the blood.

THE HEART

The heart is a cone-shaped organ about the size of a clenched fist and lies on the diaphragm, just left of the midline of the body. It provides a pumping service that maintains a constant circulation or blood flow to carry oxygen and carbon dioxide around the body. The wall of the heart is made up of three layers. The *myocardium* (*myo* meaning muscle), which is the middle layer, is the predominant layer and is essentially the heart muscle. The myocardium is covered on the inside by a layer of tissue known as the *endocardium* (*endo* meaning within) and on the outside by a layer

FIG. 7.1

The cardiopulmonary system

of tissue known as the *epicardium* (*epi* meaning without). The entire heart is then surrounded by a fibrous tissue called the *pericardium* (*peri* meaning around), which is filled with fluid in order to protect and anchor the heart.

NEED TO KNOW
The heart beats about 100,000 times a day, or 35 million times a year, and pumps blood around an estimated 100,000km of blood vessels.

The heart can be divided into left and right sides by a muscular wall known as the *septum*, which literally translates as 'dividing wall'. Each side contains an upper and a lower chamber.

Each upper chamber is called an *atrium* (*atrium* meaning entry hall) and each lower chamber is called a *ventricle* (*ventricle* meaning little belly). The left ventricle is larger and has thicker walls than the right ventricle, as it pumps blood into the arteries and has to force against the pressure of the blood exerted as the arteries become progressively smaller.

Blood flow through the heart is a one-way system controlled by a number of one-way valves. The four main valves in the heart are as follows:

- **Atrioventricular valves** The atrioventricular valves control the flow of blood between the atrium and ventricles. The right atrioventricular valve is called the *tricuspid valve* and the left is called the *bicuspid* or *mitral valve*.

- **Semilunar valves** As the name suggests, semilunar valves are in the shape of a half-moon (*semi* meaning half and *lunar* meaning moon-shaped). These valves are located at the exits to arteries from the respective ventricles. The right ventricle valve, leading to the opening of the pulmonary artery, is called the *pulmonary valve* and the left ventricle valve, leading to the opening of the aorta, is called the *aortic valve*.

NEED TO KNOW
Aorte means to suspend, as it was once thought that the job of the main artery, the aorta, was to lift up the heart.

THE CARDIAC CYCLE

All chambers of the heart contract and relax in a specific sequence in order to pump blood out or to fill up with blood. *Cardiac cycle* refers to this sequence of contraction and relaxation – in other words, the time taken from the start of one beat to the start of another beat. The cardiac cycle can be measured by a qualified person using an ECG machine, which produces a trace known as the PQRST wave. This is essentially the trace of electrical activity across the heart during the cardiac cycle. The electrical activity in the heart is activated subconsciously by the sinoatrial node, which is a group of specialised cells in the right atrium responsible for the ordered contraction and relaxation of the heart. The sinoatrial node is also known as the natural pacemaker.

NEED TO KNOW
Each heartbeat is stimulated by an electrical impulse that originates in a small strip of heart tissue known as the sinoatrial (S-A) node, or pacemaker.

One of the most important advances in cardiology is the electrical pacemaker. This originates the electrical impulses when the patient's is defective.

The sequence of electrical activity across the heart during a cardiac cycle is quite quick as the heart beats on average about 72 times per minute. The number of times the heart beats every minute is called the heart rate and is measured in beats per minute (bpm). The sequence of events for the cardiac cycle is as follows:

1. The 'P' section represents the contraction of the atria (atrial systole), which pumps blood into the ventricles. At this point, the ventricles are relaxed (ventricular diastole). Electrical activity is not very high as the atria do not contract strongly; this is because they are assisted by gravity and the blood is not under a large amount of pressure.

2. The 'QRS' section represents the forceful contraction of the ventricles (ventricular systole) to pump blood through the aortic and pulmonary valves into the respective vessels. This occurs about 0.1 seconds after the contraction of the atria. At this point, the valves between the atria and ventricles are closed to prevent backflow. The amount of blood pumped out of the ventricles each beat is called the *stroke volume* and the volume of blood left in the ventricles after they have contracted is called the *end systolic volume*.

3. The 'T' section is when the ventricles are relaxed and the atria are filling up prior to their activation. The electrical activity here is returning to a resting state.

The whole cycle lasts about 0.8 seconds.

● **Cardiac output** The amount of blood pumped out of the heart every minute is known as the cardiac output. This can be written as follows:

Cardiac output = heart rate x stroke volume

As heart rate is measured in beats per minute (bpm) and stroke volume is measured in millilitres (mls), cardiac output is measured in millilitres per minute (mls.min^{-1}). Exercise can make the heart stronger, which could result in an increase in stroke volume as the heart can pump out more blood. As sub maximal heart rate normally reduces as a long-term effect of exercise,

this would mean that even though stroke volume increases, cardiac output stays relatively the same due to the reduction in heart rate.

TASK

Give a brief description of the heart and the cardiac cycle, describing any terms that you use.

Blood

BLOOD FLOW

Two *pulmonary veins* (one from each lung) carry blood that is rich in oxygen (oxygenated blood) to the left atrium in the heart. This is known as the *pulmonary circulation system*. The blood then passes through the left atrioventricular valve into the left ventricle, from where it is forcefully pumped through the aortic valve into the first (main) artery, the *aorta*.

Oxygenated blood is then pumped around a network of arteries leading to places that require it, such as muscles and organs. This is known as the *systemic circulation system*. The oxygen is delivered into the muscles or organs through the smallest vessels, known as capillaries, and at the same time carbon dioxide passes from the muscles or organs into the capillaries. This exchange of gases is known as *diffusion*.

The deoxygenated blood then makes the return journey to the heart, carrying waste products such as carbon dioxide. The blood moves through a network of veins into the two main veins, called the *superior* and *inferior vena cavae*. These two veins empty the blood into the right atrium. The blood then passes through the right atrioventricular valve into the right ventricle. This process is called *venous return*.

The right ventricle then pumps the deoxygenated blood through the pulmonary valve and into the pulmonary artery. This leads back to the lungs, where carbon dioxide passes out of the capillaries into the lungs and oxygen is diffused back into the capillaries to be taken back to the left atrium via the pulmonary vein. The journey the blood makes from the right ventricle via the lungs to the left atrium is known as *pulmonary circulation*. The process then starts again. For more information on the function of the lungs, see chapter 8.

THE COMPOSITION OF BLOOD

Blood is made up of straw-coloured transparent fluid called *plasma* and different types of cells that are suspended in the plasma. Typically, blood contains about 55 per cent plasma and 45 per cent cells. The two types of cells within blood are known as red and white blood cells.

- **Red blood cells** Otherwise known as *erythrocytes*, red blood cells are made in the bone marrow and last for about 120 days, circulating within the body. Red blood cells contain a protein known as *haemoglobin*, which is responsible for combining with oxygen or carbon dioxide to transport it through the bloodstream. When haemoglobin combines with oxygen, it is known as *oxyhaemoglobin*; when carbon dioxide is transported in the blood, it is known as *carbaminohaemoglobin*.

- **White blood cells** Otherwise known as *leukocytes*, white blood cells are the largest of the blood cells and account for about 1 per cent of the total blood volume. The main function of white blood cells is to protect the body against any foreign bodies and to remove any waste material, called *cell debris*. There are many different types of leukocytes, which have specific roles within the body.

- **Platelets** These are very small discs made in the red bone marrow that have a lifespan of between 8 and 11 days. Platelets help to prevent

blood loss when a blood vessel is damaged. First, they are involved in vasoconstriction of the vessel at the damaged site and then in plugging the break. They are then involved in blood clotting at the site of the damage. When all of this occurs, the damage to the vessel can be repaired and breakdown of the clot can begin.

The circulation system

Within the body is a network of vessels known as arteries, veins and capillaries that carry the blood and its contents to all areas. These vessels each have different functions and structures.

ARTERIES

Arteries carry oxygenated blood that is under pressure away from the heart. Arteries are round with thick, elastic, muscular walls to withstand the pressure. Because of the muscular walls, arteries can get narrower (*vasoconstriction*) or open up (*vasodilation*). The space inside the artery is known as the *lumen*. In cases of heart disease, the lumen can become blocked by fatty deposits (*atherosclerosis*), which can then restrict blood flow and increase blood pressure. See Fig. 7.2.

Arteries close to the heart are thicker than those further away due to the increased pressure they have to withstand. As the arteries branch out away from the heart, they become smaller and are known as *arterioles*. As they branch out even further, they become minute vessels called *capillaries* (see page 104–105).

VEINS

Veins carry the blood back to the heart once it has delivered oxygen to the sites that require it. In other words, veins carry deoxygenated blood.

FIG. 7.2

A typical artery

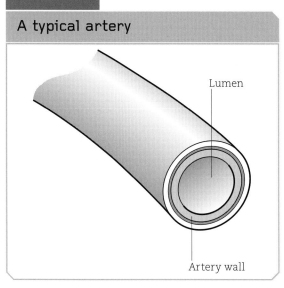

Lumen

Artery wall

The veins are not as round as arteries and have thinner walls, as there is less pressure on them. See Fig. 7.3.

FIG. 7.3

A typical vein

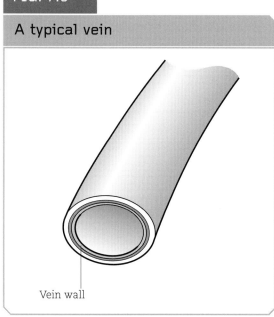

Vein wall

Oxygenated blood flows through arteries then passes into arterioles then capillaries. The deoxygenated blood (having given up its oxygen) then flows into vessels called venules, which in turn then flow into larger vessels called veins. As the blood that veins carry is not under as much pressure as that carried by the arteries, the veins need a system (known as venous return) to prevent a possible backflow of blood, which could lead to an effect called *blood pooling*, which is essentially an inefficient return of deoxygenated blood back to the heart. This would certainly reduce the capacity for exercise and might also cause dizziness and fatigue. Veins therefore have a series of one-way valves that prevent the blood from flowing backwards against the normal direction of blood flow. These one-way valves can get damaged due to high blood pressure or disease, which can have the effect of reducing venous return. Other mechanisms that contribute to venous return are gravity, muscle contraction and breathing.

- **Gravity** Any blood that is above the level of the heart is assisted by gravity to help it return to the heart.

- **Muscle contraction** Skeletal muscle contraction and smooth muscle peristaltic action help to pump blood back to the heart. For example, when we walk or run, the calf muscle contracts with heel lift, which squeezes blood from the lower extremities back towards the heart.

- **Breathing** Breathing increases pressure in the abdominal cavity, which assists blood flow back to the heart.

CAPILLARIES

Capillaries are the smallest vessels of both arteries and veins. They are only one cell thick and porous so that carbon dioxide, oxygen and other

FIG. 7.4

A typical capillary

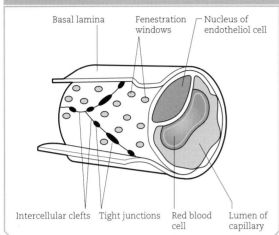

Basal lamina
Fenestration windows
Nucleus of endotheliol cell
Intercellular clefts
Tight junctions
Red blood cell
Lumen of capillary

substances can pass through in a process called *gaseous exchange*. However, red blood cells cannot pass through the capillary walls. See Fig. 7.4.

Thousands of capillaries wrap around muscles so that oxygen can be delivered and carbon dioxide extracted. At the start of a network, before they branch out, capillaries have muscular sphincters (round muscles) that can open or close to either allow or prevent blood flow to the network (sometimes called *blood shunting*). These are used to ensure the areas of the body that need it the most receive oxygen at the expense of other areas. For example, when there is an increased demand for oxygen by muscles during exercise, capillary sphincters will open at the muscles doing the exercise and close in places such as the digestive system where oxygen is not required.

TASK
Describe the composition of blood, the vessels that carry the blood and the method by which oxygen circulates around the body.

Blood pressure and exercise

Pressure is needed to pump the blood around the body otherwise it would simply gravitate to the lowest parts of the body. The pressure is greatest at the aorta, as the left ventricle forcefully pumps the blood through it. By the time the blood reaches the capillaries, it is still under pressure, but not as much as in the aorta.

There are two phases of blood pressure: *systolic* and *diastolic*. Systolic pressure is the pressure on the artery walls when the ventricles contract and diastolic pressure is the pressure on the artery walls when the ventricles fill between beats.

The two phases of pressure can be measured to evaluate if an individual is within safe limits. Blood pressure is measured in millimetres of mercury (mmHg). The American College of Sports Medicine recommends that an average of two or more readings be taken when testing blood pressure. Table 7.1 shows the ranges for normal and high blood pressure.

If blood pressure goes above or below the normal range, it is deemed to be high or low respectively. High blood pressure is known as *hypertension* and low blood pressure is known as *hypotension*. Even though physical activity is recommended for hypertensive people it must be mentioned that during any form of physical exertion blood pressure can in fact increase. Blood pressure can change during both resistance training and aerobic-type activity. For example, it is generally accepted that during aerobic-type activities, systolic blood pressure increases as the work being done increases whereas diastolic pressure usually remains about the same or in some instances can actually become lower. There is a great deal of evidence that suggests that an exaggerated blood pressure response when testing during aerobic activity may be an indication of future hypertension and even

TABLE 7.1

Ranges for normal and high blood pressure (in mmHg)

	Systolic	Diastolic
Hypotension	<90	<60
Normal	<120 and	<80
Pre-hypertension	120–139 or	80–89
Hypertension (stage 1)	140–159 or	90–99
Hypertension (stage 2)	≥160–179 or	≥100–109

Adapted from the ACSM GETP (2018)

myocardial infarction. There are, however, problems associated with the measurement of blood pressure during any type of activity. For example, although systolic blood pressure can be recorded reasonably well during bicycle exercise, it is often the case that diastolic values are overestimated or underestimated. Much research has also been done on the response of blood pressure to resistance training. It has been demonstrated that blood pressure can rise to 400/300 mmHg during maximum heavy resistance training; therefore this type of training is obviously not recommended for those with hypertension. Fig. 7.5 shows typical systolic and diastolic pressure changes during aerobic activity.

It can be seen in Fig. 7.5 that arm exercises (small muscle groups) can have a greater effect on blood pressure than larger muscle group exercises. Note also that the diastolic blood pressure is at or even below resting levels following large muscle group aerobic exercises. It should also be emphasised that as blood pressure can increase during exercise, no exercise should be done if resting systolic pressure is above 200mmHg or diastolic pressure is above 110mmHg.

HYPERTENSION

High blood pressure can be caused by various factors, but regardless of the cause, the rate of the heart and force at which it contracts are increased to maintain the amount of blood required by the body. Long-term hypertension can result in heart attack or stroke.

FIG. 7.5

Typical systolic and diastolic pressure changes during aerobic activity

During a bout of exercise, systolic blood pressure tends to rise whereas diastolic blood pressure stays about the same (and can even decrease slightly). Regular low-intensity aerobic exercise has been shown to reduce both systolic and diastolic blood pressure. Exercise can also prevent the tendency for blood pressure to rise in the long term. This preventative measure is important, as there is less risk of heart disease in individuals who have never been hypertensive.

HYPOTENSION

Hypotension refers to blood pressure below the normal range. Although the effects are not the same as in hypertension, individuals who have lower than normal blood pressure should be advised to move slowly when coming from a floor position to a standing position. This is because the low blood pressure can cause a reduction in blood flow to the brain due to gravity, which can cause fainting.

NEED TO KNOW

People with hypertension should avoid isometric or heavy resistance exercises as they can elevate blood pressure. Also, trying to perform an exercise while attempting a forceful exhalation against a closed airway (glottis) is not recommended as this could cause an increase in blood pressure. This is known as the *Valsalva manoeuvre*.

The effects of exercise on the heart

SHORT-TERM EFFECTS

Exercise leads to an increase in the rate of *cardiac output* (CO). The stroke volume is also increased, as the heart is pumping faster to supply oxygenated blood to the working muscles.

LONG-TERM EFFECTS

The long-term effects of exercise on the heart include the following:

1. An increase in the size and strength of the cardiac muscle.
2. An increase in venous return, which reduces blood pooling.
3. Working (systolic) and resting (diastolic) blood pressure lowers, enabling the heart to work more efficiently.
4. The resting and sub-maximal heart rate decreases.
5. Stroke volume increases.
6. The heart adapts to bouts of physical activity through hypertrophy (increase in size). This makes the individual more efficient at providing blood to the muscles during physical activity.

The effects of exercise on the circulation system

SHORT-TERM EFFECTS

The short-term effects of exercise on the circulation system include the following:

1. Blood is diverted from non-essential areas (for example, the digestive system) to the muscles that are being used.
2. Some blood vessels narrow (vasoconstrict) and some widen (vasodilate).

LONG-TERM EFFECTS

The long-term effects of exercise on the circulation system include the following:

1. An improvement in general circulation.
2. Vasoconstriction and vasodilation become more efficient.
3. The number of capillaries and mitochondria increases.

4. Greater quantities of red blood cells are produced in order to meet the requirements for an increase in the oxygen-carrying capacity of the blood.
5. There are increased levels of haemoglobin in the blood to increase the blood's capacity to bind and transport oxygen to the working muscles.

TABLE 7.2

Cardiovascular differences between population groups

Population group	Main cardiovascular differences	Exercise implication
Children/ young people	Walking/running economy is less Cardiac output and stroke volume lower Thermoregulation not as efficient Higher maximum heart rate	Perform extended warm-up/cool-downs and limit duration of higher intensity activities Avoid extremes of temperature and keep well hydrated, especially in winter Always supervise exercises
Older adults	Cardiac output, stroke volume, VO_2 max and heart rate decrease Blood pressure increases	Any progression should be slow and to individual capacity Get regular feedback during and after exercise Introduce post-exercise relaxation Avoid fatigue Use cycling and swimming for those with reduced weight-bearing capacity
Ante-/post- natal	Increase in resting heart rate Decrease in venous return Cardiac output increases Left ventricle and blood vessels enlarge Blood flow to the skin increases	Avoid exercises in the supine position Be aware of heating up quickly Limit higher intensity to short periods No high impact and no exhaustion Low intensity only (after medical approval) if there is no history of exercise Stop if any pain or discomfort

Key cardiovascular differences between various population groups

Instructors should be aware that there are cardiovascular differences between an apparently healthy population and population groups (children/young people, older adults and ante-/postnatal). Table 7.2 outlines the main differences and the implications for exercise.

EXAMPLE QUESTIONS

7.1 The heart muscle is divided into left and right sides by what?

   a) endocardium

   b) epicardium

   c) mitrum

   d) septum

7.2 The heart muscle is entirely covered by a layer of fibrous tissue known as what?

   a) pericardium

   b) epicardium

   c) endocardium

   d) myocardium

7.3 The term 'entry hall' relates to which structure in the heart?

   a) sino-atrial node

   b) ventricle

   c) atrium

   d) aorta

7.4 The mitral valve is otherwise known as the what?

   a) aortic

   b) tri-cuspid

   c) bi-cuspid

   d) semilunar

7.5 The sino-atrial node can be found in which chamber of the heart?

   a) right atrium

   b) left atrium

   c) right ventricle

   d) left ventricle

7.6 The aortic valve can be found leading from which chamber of the heart?

   a) right atrium

   b) left atrium

   c) right ventricle

   d) left ventricle

7.7 The amount of blood pumped out of the ventricles each beat is known as what?

a) end diastolic volume

b) cardiac output

c) stroke volume

d) residual volume

7.8 The amount of blood pumped out of the ventricles each beat, multiplied by the heart rate in beats per minute is known as what?

a) end diastolic volume

b) cardiac output

c) stroke volume

d) residual volume

7.9 The amount of blood left in the ventricles after each beat is known as what?

a) end diastolic volume

b) cardiac output

c) stroke volume

d) residual volume

7.10 Which of the following protect the body against foreign bodies?

a) white blood cells

b) red blood cells

c) plasma

d) platelets

7.11 Which of the following help in blood clotting?

a) red blood cells

b) platelets

c) plasma

d) white blood cells

7.12 Blood pressure is greatest in which vessel?

a) pulmonary artery

b) pulmonary vein

c) aorta

d) vena cava

Further reading

Abrahams, P., Craven, J. and Lumley, J. (2011) *Illustrated Clinical Anatomy* (2nd ed.), Hodder Arnold

American College of Obstetricians and Gynecologists (2002) 'ACOG Committee Opinion No.267: Exercise during pregnancy and the postpartum period', *Obstetrics and Gynecology*, 99: 171–173

American College of Sports Medicine (2018) *Guidelines to Exercise Testing and Prescription* (10th ed.), Lippincott, Williams & Wilkins

American Congress of Obstetricians and Gynecologists (2003) *Exercise During Pregnancy*, ACOG

Baechle, R.T. (2016) *Essentials of Strength Training and Conditioning* (4th ed.), Human Kinetics

Fitzgerald, M.D., Tanaka, H., Tran, Z.V. and Seals, D.R. (1997) 'Age-related declines in maximal aerobic capacity in regularly exercising vs. sedentary women: a meta-analysis', *Journal of Applied Physiology*, 83: 160–165

Kubukeli, Z.N., Noakes, T.D. and Dennis, S.C. (2002) 'Training techniques to improve endurance exercise performances', *Sports Medicine* 32: 489–509

Marieb, E.N. and Hoehn, K. (2019) *Human Anatomy and Physiology* (11th ed.), Pearson

McArdle, W.D., Katch, F.I. and Katch, V.L. (2015) *Exercise Physiology* (8th ed.), Lippincott, Williams & Wilkins

Paisley, T.S., Joy, E.A. and Price, R.J. (2003) 'Exercise during pregnancy: a practical approach', *Current Sports Medicine Reports*, 2: 325–330

Pendergast, D.R., Fisher, N.M. and Calkins, E. (1993) 'Cardiovascular, neuromuscular and metabolic alterations with age leading to frailty', *Journal of Gerontology*, 48: 61–67

Porter, S. (2008) *The Anatomy Workbook* (2nd ed.), Butterworth Heinemann

Ross, J.S. and Wilson, J.W. (2018) *Anatomy and Physiology in Health and Illness* (13th ed.), Churchill Livingstone

Sewell, D., Watkins, P. and Griffin, M. (2012) *Sport and Exercise Science: An introduction* (2nd ed.), Hodder Arnold.

Tortora, G.J. and Grabowski, S.R. (2017) *Principles of Anatomy and Physiology* (15th ed.), Wiley

Twisk, J. (2001) 'Physical activity guidelines for children and adolescents: a critical review', *Sports Medicine*, 31: 617–627

Kenney, L., Wilmore, J.H. and Costhill, D.L. (2019) *Physiology of Sport and Exercise* (7th ed.), Human Kinetics.

The Respiratory System

OBJECTIVES

After completing this chapter, you will be able to:

1 Describe the structure of the lungs in relation to their function.
2 Explain the passage of air into and out of the lungs.
3 Explain the process of exchange of gases.
4 List the percentages of gases in inspired and expired air.
5 Explain the mechanism of breathing.
6 Explain the short- and long-term effects of exercise on the respiratory system.
7 Describe the key respiratory differences in various population groups.

Introduction

This chapter deals with the anatomical system of the body in relation to the respiratory system from the perspective of structure, function and the effects of exercise. Within the Professional Standards framework, instructors should be able to describe the common structures of the respiratory system and describe the function of the system, as well as describe how exercise can impact on the system.

Later chapters in the book provide physiological and biomechanical principles that, together with the knowledge of the cardiovascular system covered in the previous chapter and the respiratory system covered in this chapter, provide you with the understanding and ability to design appropriate exercise programmes for apparently healthy individuals

and to understand the effects of various types of exercise on the human body.

The respiratory system

The *respiratory system* is the collective term given to the nose, pharynx, larynx, trachea, bronchi and lungs. Essentially, it filters, warms and moistens air before conducting it to the lungs, which house specific sites where gases are exchanged between the air and the blood. See Fig. 8.1.

THE LUNGS

The lungs are a pair of cone-shaped organs made of elastic tissue that expand to allow

FIG. 8.1

The respiratory system

THE PASSAGE OF AIR

air from the atmosphere to enter. They are roughly level with the heart in the thoracic cavity and are surrounded by a double membrane called the *pleura*. Each lung has a superior (upper), middle and inferior (lower) lobe.

THE PASSAGE OF AIR

Air that is breathed in is known as *inspired air*, while air that is breathed out is called *expired air*. Air is made up of various gases, and the composition of gases in inspired air is different to that of expired air (see Table 8.1). About 5 per cent of the oxygen in inspired air is used up, so expired air contains less oxygen. About 4 per cent carbon dioxide is produced during breathing, so expired air has more carbon dioxide than inspired air.

The *passage of air* describes how oxygen from the air reaches the muscles that require it for the production of energy. First, air is taken

TABLE 8.1

Composition of inspired and expired air*

	Inspired air (%)	Expired air (%)
Oxygen	21	16
Carbon dioxide	0.04	4
Nitrogen	78	78

*approximate due to trace gases

in through the mouth or the nose. If the air is passed through the nose, it can be warmed, moistened and filtered; this occurs to a lesser extent to air taken in through the mouth, which can induce asthmatic reactions. The air then passes through the *pharynx* (throat), which lies behind the nose and the mouth and is a passage for food and air. The pharynx is lined with a mucous membrane that provides moisture, and the wall of the pharynx is made of skeletal muscle. The pharynx also houses the tonsils, which play a part in reactions against foreign invaders such as viruses.

The air then passes down through the *larynx* (voice box), which extends to the level of the start of the thoracic vertebrae. The air is continually warmed and moistened as it travels through the larynx. The larynx wall is made up of several pieces of cartilage connected by muscle tissue. One of the pieces of cartilage is known as the *epiglottis* (*epi* meaning over and *glottis* meaning tongue), which is essentially a trapdoor that controls the passage of air and food (it closes when swallowing to prevent food and drink going into the airways). From the larynx, the air continues into a rigid cartilaginous tube called the *trachea* (*trachea* meaning sturdy) or windpipe, which is lined with fine hairs that filter the air. The trachea runs down to the level of the fifth thoracic vertebra, where it divides into the left and right *bronchi*.

NEED TO KNOW
The thyroid cartilage is a small piece of cartilage at the front of the throat, otherwise known as the Adam's apple. Its role is to influence the tension of the vocal cords and is usually larger in males, which is why men have deeper voices than women.

Air passes into each of the bronchi, which enter the left and right lungs and split into smaller bronchi. These then split into smaller tubes called *bronchioles*, which in turn branch out and finally lead into air sacs called *alveoli*. The alveoli then fill up with air and expand to a size dependent on breathing levels and other physical factors.

It is here that gaseous exchange takes place, so that oxygen can enter the bloodstream to be transported to working muscles and carbon dioxide can be removed from the bloodstream in expired air. The amount of air remaining in the lungs after a maximal breath out is known as the *residual volume*.

NEED TO KNOW
Sometimes the airflow through the trachea can become blocked. Therefore, an incision is made through the wall of the trachea and a tube inserted so that the patient can breathe. This serious medical procedure is known as a tracheotomy.

GASEOUS EXCHANGE

In order for oxygen to pass from the alveoli into the bloodstream, it must first pass through the walls of the alveoli. All alveoli are surrounded by numerous capillaries, which then lead into the network of veins and arteries. Oxygen can pass through the membrane wall of the alveoli and through the wall of the capillaries, as both structures are only one cell thick. Carbon dioxide passes the opposite way, from the capillaries into the alveoli, to be breathed out (see Fig. 8.2.).

This exchange of gases is possible due to the *pressure gradient*. In general terms, gases pass from an area of high concentration (or pressure) to an area of low concentration in order to

FIG. 8.2

Gaseous exchange at the alveoli

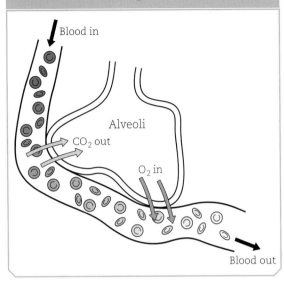

Blood in

Alveoli

CO_2 out

O_2 in

Blood out

equalise the concentration. For example, after breathing in (*inspiration*) there is a higher concentration of oxygen in the alveoli than in the capillaries surrounding them, so the oxygen diffuses from the alveoli to the capillaries. Likewise, there is a higher concentration of carbon dioxide in the capillaries than in the alveoli, so the carbon dioxide diffuses from the capillaries into the alveoli.

BREATHING CONTROL

Breathing is more technically known as ventilation. One of the main factors involved in breathing control is the level of carbon dioxide in the blood. When the amount of carbon dioxide in the blood reaches a certain level, respiratory centres in the brainstem activate breathing muscles via the central nervous system.

Generally, the breathing rate (the number of breaths per minute) is about 12 times per minute. This increases during exercise, as the demand for more oxygen by the working muscles is recognised by the respiratory centre in the brainstem, which in turn increases the number of breaths per minute. Therefore, in this way the breathing rate is controlled subconsciously. Breathing can also be controlled consciously.

The amount of air taken into the lungs during a normal breath is called the *tidal volume*. The maximum amount of air breathed out after a maximal inspiration is called the *vital capacity* and is sometimes measured to monitor progress during an exercise programme although it is mainly used to identify possible lung disease.

THE ROLE OF MUSCLES IN BREATHING

The main muscles involved in breathing in (inspiration) when an individual is not involved in exercise are the diaphragm and the external intercostals. The scalenes and the pectoralis minor contribute during vigorous exercise. Essentially when the inspiratory muscles contract, the diaphragm has the effect of pulling the ribcage down and expanding the thorax area, which results in drawing air in as the pressure of the lungs that have stretched is less than the air pressure outside the body. This is called a pressure gradient.

Expiration (breathing out) is predominantly passive, as the result of *elastic recoil* by certain tissues: tissues such as muscles have a certain amount of elasticity, which means they will return to their pre-stretched state when the contraction stops. The muscles involved in expiration are the internal intercostals and certain abdominal muscles. During forced expiration (breathing heavily), the transversus abdominis is also used.

THE MECHANICS OF BREATHING (VENTILATION)

There are several steps that occur during ventilation:

- At the start of inspiration the phrenic nerve stimulates the diaphragm and external intercostal muscles to contract.
- Upon contraction, the diaphragm descends downwards and the external intercostal muscles elevate the ribs upwards and outwards. This enlarges the volume of the thoracic cavity, as can be seen in Fig. 8.3a.
- As the thoracic cavity enlarges, the lungs are forced to expand to fill the larger thoracic cavity.
- The pressure within the alveoli drops below that of the atmosphere as the air molecules occupy a larger lung volume, resulting in air flow into the lungs (this is often referred to as 'airflow down the pressure gradient').
- The air continues to enter the lung until the pressure inside the lungs is the same as the atmosphere (in other words, no pressure gradient).

- At this point the inspiratory muscles relax.
- As the lungs have an elastic property they recoil and become smaller in volume, which increases the alveolar pressure.
- The pressure inside the lungs is now higher than the atmosphere so air now travels from the lungs into the atmosphere until the pressure is equal, as shown in Fig. 8.3b. The cycle then restarts.

TYPICAL LUNG VOLUME AND CAPACITY

There are many factors that can affect lung volume and capacity, such as genetics, gender and body size. Volume is the measure of a single function, such as breathing in, whereas capacity is the measure of more than one function. Volume is typically divided into 4 areas or units:

FIG. 8.3

(a) Inhalation (b) Exhalation

Air inhaled

Rib cage expands as rib muscles contract

Lung

Diaphragm

INHALATION
diaphragm contracts
(moves down)

Air exhaled

Rib cage gets smaller as rib muscles relax

EXHALATION
diaphragm relaxes
(moves up)

1. *Tidal volume (TV)* – this is a measure of the air that is inspired and expired during a normal breath. This is usually in the region of 50 ml (half a litre).
2. *Expiratory Reserve Volume (ERV)* – this is the additional amount of air that could be exhaled after a normal breath.
3. *Inspiratory Reserve Volume (IRV)* – this is the additional amount of air that could be inhaled after a normal breath.
4. *Residual Volume (RV)* – this is the air left in the lungs after the ERV is exhaled.

Lung volumes and capacities are measured by a technique known as spirometry. One of the most common capacity measures is Forced Vital Capacity (FVC), which is the total amount of air that can be forcibly exhaled after a maximal breath in. An average person has a lung capacity of about 6 litres; however, we rarely operate at full capacity.

NEED TO KNOW

The largest lung capacity ever recorded was more than 11 litres!

TASK

List and describe the structures of the respiratory system and explain how oxygen and carbon dioxide are exchanged between the air and the blood.

TABLE 8.2

Respiratory differences between population groups

Population group	Main cardiovascular differences	Exercise implication
Children/young people	Higher breathing rate (ventilation)	Children have to breathe faster for any given intensity so reduce the duration of high-intensity exercise
Older adults	Lung capacity and forced expiratory volume decrease due to muscle weakness and loss of alveoli elasticity Maximal ventilation decreases	Reduce intensity of exercise due to shortness of breath
Ante-/postnatal	Higher breathing rate (ventilation) as a result of increased sensitivity to carbon dioxide Decreased residual volume Increased oxygen consumption Hyperventilation can occur	Reduce intensity of exercise due to shortness of breath (even at low intensity) Be aware that hyperventilation can occur

The effects of smoking on the respiratory system

The exact mechanisms of the effects of smoking on the respiratory system are complicated and are still being investigated in current research. However, a summary of the effects is given below:

1. Tar from cigarettes can remain in the alveoli, which can restrict the amount of air taken in.
2. Cigarette smoke can destroy the alveoli wall, which prevents the diffusion of oxygen and carbon dioxide.
3. Smoking is one of the leading causes of chronic bronchitis, which is the inflammation of the airways leading to a restriction in the passage of air.
4. Smoking is one of the most common causes of lung cancer. Most people with lung cancer die within the first year of diagnosis.
5. Pneumonia, which relates to inflammation of the alveoli, can be caused by smoking.
6. Nicotine from cigarettes narrows the smaller airways, which can decrease the airflow.
7. Haemoglobin (the oxygen carrier in the blood) prefers to carry carbon monoxide from smoke rather than oxygen, which reduces its oxygen-carrying capacity.
8. Smoking can cause increased mucous secretion and destroy the lining of the airways.

The effects of exercise on the respiratory system

SHORT-TERM EFFECTS

The short-term effects of exercise on the respiratory system include the following:

1. The rate of exchange of gases within the lungs increases, as does the volume of gases exchanged.
2. Levels of carbon dioxide in the body increase, so more has to be removed.
3. The depth of breathing increases, followed by the rate of breathing.

LONG-TERM EFFECTS

The long-term effects of exercise on the respiratory system include the following:

1. The respiratory muscles become stronger.
2. Gaseous exchange at the alveoli takes place more easily.
3. The breathing effort required decreases.
4. The number of capillaries increases.
5. Tidal volume and vital capacity can increase.

Key respiratory differences between various population groups

Instructors should be aware that there are respiratory differences between an apparently healthy population and various population groups (children/young people, older adults and ante-/postnatal). Table 8.2 outlines the main differences and the implications for exercise.

EXAMPLE QUESTIONS

8.1 What structures lead directly into the alveoli?

a) bronchioles

b) pleura

c) capillaries

d) bronchi

8.2 The double membrane surrounding the lungs is known as what?

a) alveoli

b) pleura

c) bronchioles

d) capillaries

8.3 The passage of oxygen and carbon dioxide in and out of the alveoli is known as what?

a) gaseous exchange

b) pressure gradient

c) elastic recoil

d) passage of air

8.4 What is the percentage of oxygen in the air that is inspired?

a) 17

b) 5

c) 21

d) 78

8.5 The amount of air left in the lungs after a breath out is known as what?

a) expiratory ratio

b) tidal volume

c) residual volume

d) vital capacity

8.6 The maximum amount of air breathed out of the lungs after a maximum breath in is known as what?

a) expiratory ratio

b) tidal volume

c) residual volume

d) vital capacity

8.7 Which of the following gases stimulates breathing when blood levels reach a certain point?

    a) oxygen

    b) carbon dioxide

    c) nitrogen

    d) hydrogen

8.8 The amount of air taken into the lungs during a normal breath is called what?

    a) expiratory ratio

    b) tidal volume

    c) residual volume

    d) vital capacity

8.9 Smoking is thought to be one of the main causes of what?

    a) chronic bronchitis

    b) heart attack

    c) high cholesterol

    d) obesity

8.10 Inflammation of the alveoli is otherwise known as what?

    a) emphysema

    b) bronchitis

    c) pneumonia

    d) pleurisy

8.11 Normal expiration is brought about as a result of what effect?

    a) muscle contraction

    b) gaseous exchange

    c) pressure gradient

    d) elastic recoil

8.12 Which is the main muscle involved in forced expiration?

    a) multifidus

    b) rectus abdominis

    c) diaphragm

    d) transversus abdominis

Further reading

Abrahams, P., Craven, J. and Lumley, J. (2011) *Illustrated Clinical Anatomy* (2nd ed.), Hodder Arnold

American College of Obstetricians and Gynecologists (2002) 'ACOG Committee Opinion No.267: Exercise during pregnancy and the postpartum period', *Obstetrics and Gynecology*, 99: 171–173

American Congress of Obstetricians and Gynecologists (2003) *Exercise During Pregnancy*, ACOG

Baechle, R.T. (2016) *Essentials of Strength Training and Conditioning* (4th ed.), Human Kinetics

Fitzgerald, M.D., Tanaka, H., Tran, Z.V. and Seals, D.R. (1997) 'Age-related declines in maximal aerobic capacity in regularly exercising vs. sedentary women: a meta-analysis', *Journal of Applied Physiology*, 83: 160–165

Marieb, E.N. and Hoehn, K. (2019) *Human Anatomy and Physiology* (11th ed.), Pearson

McArdle, W.D., Katch, F.I. and Katch, V.L. (2015) *Exercise Physiology* (8th ed.), Lippincott, Williams & Wilkins

Paisley, T.S., Joy, E.A. and Price, R.J. (2003) 'Exercise during pregnancy: a practical approach', *Current Sports Medicine Reports*, 2: 325–330

Porter, S. (2008) *The Anatomy Workbook* (2nd ed.), Butterworth Heinemann

Ross, J.S. and Wilson, J.W. (2018) *Anatomy and Physiology in Health and Illness* (13th ed.), Churchill Livingstone

Sewell, D., Watkins, P. and Griffin, M. (2012) *Sport and Exercise Science: An Introduction* (2nd ed.), Hodder Arnold

Tortora, G.J. and Grabowski, S.R. (2017) *Principles of Anatomy and Physiology* (15th ed.), Wiley

Twisk, J. (2001) 'Physical activity guidelines for children and adolescents: a critical review', *Sports Medicine*, 31: 617–627

Kenney, L., Wilmore, J.H. and Costhill, D.L. (2019) *Physiology of Sport and Exercise* (7th ed.), Human Kinetics

9 Core Stability

OBJECTIVES

After completing this chapter, you will be able to:

1   Define the terms 'stabiliser' and 'mobiliser' in relation to muscle roles.
2   Identify muscles known as local and global.
3   List the methods of spinal stabilisation.
4   Define 'neutral zone' and explain the teaching methods related to this.
5   Explain the principle of intra-abdominal pressure.
6   Describe the process for the contraction of the transversus abdominis.
7   List and describe common stability exercises.
8   Discuss exercise guidelines related to core stability.

Introduction

This chapter deals with the anatomical system of the body, in particular the structure and function of muscles associated with spinal stability. The chapter also deals with commonly prescribed exercises for short- and long-term development of the associated muscles. Within the Professional Standards framework, instructors should be able to identify the muscular system associated with spinal, or core, stabilisation and describe their functions, as well as describe how exercise can impact on efficiency and development.

Other chapters in the book provide some of the physiological and biomechanical principles that, together with the specific theory covered in this chapter, will provide you with the understanding and ability to design appropriate exercise programmes for apparently healthy individuals and to understand the effects of various types of exercise on the human body.

Core stability

In simple terms, core stability is the process of holding the shoulder and pelvic girdles (that is the centre part or core of the body) stable in order to support the movement forces from the arms and legs, which in turn will also increase the ability to balance. In order to do this, the muscles that are responsible for the stabilising role must function correctly so that the muscles responsible for movement are able to perform their function correctly. Unfortunately, in many people the muscles responsible for stabilising and movement have become less than efficient due to a number of factors, including poor posture. Everyday tasks such as sitting in cars, at desks and on sofas have led to the stabilising muscles becoming weaker, as the objects we sit on take on the role of stabilising and support. Evidence has shown that as a result, other muscles that are usually associated with movement tasks take on the role of stabilisation. This can lead to weakness in certain movements and can eventually cause muscle, tendon or ligament injury, especially in cases where the speed of a movement is increased. In turn, this will increase the possibility of injury due to the greater demand for stabilisation.

NEED TO KNOW
Everybody is capable of a certain degree of core stabilisation. However, in most cases specific muscles need to be re-trained to perform the role that they are physiologically best suited for.

STABILISERS AND MOBILISERS

The everyday demands placed on the posture and control of the human body mean that the muscles responsible for core stabilisation (*stabilisers*; also known as *tonic muscles*) are designed to perform endurance tasks rather than short-term or explosive tasks. These muscles are sometimes described as 'nature's corset' and are required to carry out a stabilising role for long periods of time. Due to the demands of these endurance-type tasks, stabilisers are predominantly made up of type I slow-twitch fibres (see pages 42–45).

In someone with normal muscular function, while the role of stabilisation is being undertaken, muscles known as *mobilisers* are able to carry out their role of locomotion or movement of the body. These muscles are

usually required to provide a short-term or *phasic* role, and are therefore not classed as endurance muscles. Mobiliser muscles are predominantly made up of fast-twitch fibres and are more superficial (closer to the surface) than stabiliser muscles. Table 9.1 lists the muscles that are commonly associated with either stabilisation or mobilisation at the core, hip and shoulder.

It is commonplace for stabilising and mobilising muscles to be trained in the opposite role from that which they were designed for. For example, the rectus abdominis is predominantly a fast-twitch muscle close to the surface of the body and is normally active in strength or explosive tasks, such as running and jumping where the legs come towards the torso (spinal flexion). However, it is common for exercise programmes to include sit-up type exercises that are performed repetitively in an endurance-type capacity. The rectus abdominis is mainly responsible for this sit-up action, which effectively results in a predominantly fast-twitch muscle taking on the role of a slow-twitch muscle. This often weakens the stabiliser muscles, as the rectus abdominis has taken on this role. The drawback of this is that the rectus abdominis tries to perform both stabilising and mobilising roles, potentially leading to back pain or injury as optimal stabilisation of the spine is not performed. This reversal of roles is a common problem in exercise programmes for many different muscles within the body.

NEED TO KNOW
Lack of (or too much) flexibility in muscles can also affect their ability to either stabilise or mobilise.

INNER AND OUTER UNITS

Current research seems to suggest that both deep and superficial muscles in the trunk and

TABLE 9.1

Muscles associated with stabilisation and mobilisation

Area of stabilisation	Main stabiliser muscles
Core or trunk area	Stabiliser muscles with little mobilisation ability: • Transversus abdominis • Multifidus • Pelvic floor • Diaphragm • Internal obliques • Quadratus lumborum Muscles with a greater mobilisation ability: • Rectus abdominis • External oblique • Erector spinae
Hip	Stabiliser muscles with little mobilisation ability: • Gluteus medius and minimus • Piriformis • Gemellus (inferior and superior) • Obturator (internus and externus) • Quadratus femorus Muscles with a greater mobilisation ability: • Gluteus maximus • Iliopsoas • Tensor fasciae latae • Hamstrings • Adductors • Rectus femoris
Shoulder	Provides stabilisation mainly of the scapula: • Rhomboid • Trapezius • Serratus anterior • Subscapularis Provides stabilisation mainly of the humeral head: • Infraspinatus • Teres minor/major • Supraspinatus

pelvic region contribute in some way to spinal stabilisation (Richardson et al., 2003). What is not clear is the extent to which the general population has limited function of one or both of the systems.

Muscles in the body that are deep are sometimes referred to as *local muscles* or, in relation to core stabilisation, as the *inner unit*. The transversus abdominis, multifidus, pelvic floor, diaphragm and internal obliques are all examples of local muscles. Muscles that are superficial are commonly known as *global muscles* or the *outer unit*. The rectus abdominis, external obliques and some parts of the erector spinae are all global muscles. At the hip joint, the gluteus maximus and gluteus minimus are usually considered to be mobilisers and the gluteus medius is normally considered to be a stabiliser. There are many other muscles associated with stabilisation of the hip complex, but the main ones are mentioned above. The main muscles of the inner unit are listed below.

- **Transversus abdominis** This muscle forms a belt or corset around the trunk region and lies deep below the rectus abdominis muscle, which is associated with the 'six-pack'. Imagine a belt running underneath the navel, right around the body. This is the transversus abdominis muscle. See Fig. 9.1.

- **Multifidus** This is a series of many small muscles that attach between each vertebra of the spine (see Fig. 9.2). These muscles act as a kind of lashing for the bones in the spine to prevent any excessive movement.

- **Internal obliques** These attach from the lower ribs and insert into the pubic bone, and lie at an angle just above and below the navel (see Fig. 9.3). They are quite deep and cannot be seen superficially.

- **Pelvic floor** The pelvic floor muscles run from the coccyx (bones at the bottom of the spine), under the crotch area to the pubic bone at the front (see Fig. 9.4).

FIG. 9.1

Lateral view of the transversus abdominis

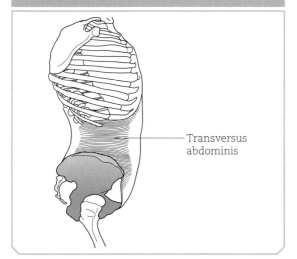

Transversus abdominis

FIG. 9.2

Posterior view of the multifidus

Multifidus

FIG. 9.3

Lateral view of the internal obliques

Internal obliques

FIG. 9.5

Anterior view of the diaphragm

is responsible for helping in breathing movements.

The inner unit or local muscles are predominantly slow-twitch (tonic) and are responsible for stabilising the core of the body, in particular the spine. The outer unit or global muscles are predominantly fast-twitch (phasic) and are mainly responsible for movement, although they do contribute in a limited way to stabilisation. The main muscles of the outer unit are described below.

- **Diaphragm**   This is a dome-shaped muscle that covers the region under the ribcage (see Fig. 9.5). As well as performing core stabilisation tasks, the diaphragm

- **Rectus abdominis**   This muscle runs the length of the abdomen from the ribs down to the pubic bone and is held in place by fascia running horizontally across the muscle which gives it the appearance of having sections (see Fig. 9.6).

FIG. 9.4

The pelvic floor muscles

Bowel

Womb

Bladder

Pubic bone

Pelvic floor muscles

- **Erector spinae**   This essentially is a group of individual muscles that run either side of the spine from the sacrum and iliac crest to the base of the skull (see Fig. 9.7).

FIG. 9.6

Anterior view of the rectus abdominis

FIG. 9.7

Posterior view of the erector spinae

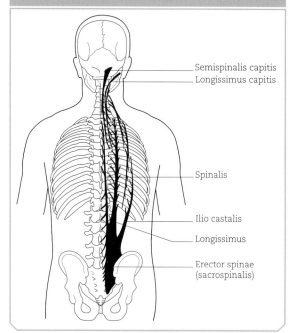

- Semispinalis capitis
- Longissimus capitis
- Spinalis
- Ilio castalis
- Longissimus
- Erector spinae (sacrospinalis)

• **External obliques** This superficial muscle lies almost at a vertical angle and runs from the surface of the lower 8 ribs down to the iliac crest (see Fig. 9.8).

In order for the spine to remain protected at all times, it is essential that both the inner and outer units are working optimally. The ability of both units to function correctly is somewhat dependent on information relayed by the neuromuscular system. If this is not functioning optimally, the inner and outer units will not function optimally. Table 9.2 provides an overview of common local and global muscles and their characteristics.

TASK

Give a brief definition of the term 'core stabilisation' and describe the differences between stabilising and mobilising muscles in relation to inner and outer units.

Mechanisms of stabilisation

The mechanisms of stabilisation of the spine (core stability) are not fully understood,

FIG. 9.8

Lateral view of the external obliques

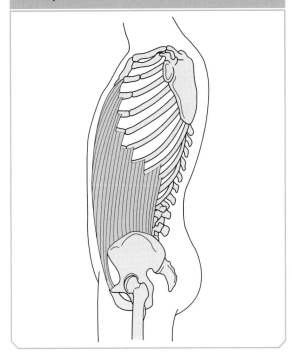

but it is thought that several systems, in conjunction with the ligaments of the spine, contribute to its overall stabilisation (although there is a body of evidence that disputes this). Systems such as *intra-abdominal pressure*, *thoraco-lumbar fascia gain* and the *hydraulic amplifier effect* are thought to provide enough spinal stabilisation for the body to carry out normal daily tasks. However, while the spine and its stabilisation systems are capable of protecting the spine under normal circumstances, an overload due to certain exercises, sport or poor posture can lead to a dysfunction in one or more of the systems, which could in turn lead to injury or postural problems (see chapter 1 for common spinal injuries and postural problems).

INTRA-ABDOMINAL PRESSURE

In order to achieve an effective degree of core stability, the stabilising muscles of the inner unit must activate and contract together to help make the trunk more solid. This can be achieved in a number of ways, one of which is a process called intra-abdominal pressure.

TABLE 9.2

Common characteristics of local and global muscles

	Local muscles (transversus abdominis, multifidus, pelvic floor, diaphragm, internal obliques)	Global muscles (rectus abdominis, external obliques, erector spinae)
Main fibre type	Slow-twitch	Fast-twitch
General task	Postural/endurance	Strength/explosive
Location	Deep	Superficial
Role	Stabilising	Mobilising
Common contraction	Isometric	Eccentric and concentric

The contents of the trunk area, including the stomach, intestines and various organs and fluid, are collectively termed the *abdominal ball* or *fluid ball*, which is cylinder-like in shape. When the core muscles contract, the walls of the abdominal ball are tightened and compressed. This creates an increase in pressure known as intra-abdominal pressure. This pushes against the spine and prevents it from making any excessive movements, and helps to keep the spine in the correct posture.

The example of an airbag inflated in a driver's seat can help to explain the process. It is difficult for the driver to move against the airbag as the pressure resists his or her movement. The same principle applies with intra-abdominal pressure, where the abdominal ball resists the movements of the spine. In effect, this encourages the spine to move as a complete unit and prevents one part of the spine moving across another part of the spine, which could easily lead to injury.

The main muscles responsible for intra-abdominal pressure are: the transversus abdominis, the internal obliques and the multifidus muscles, which form the walls of the abdominal ball; the diaphragm, which forms the top of the abdominal ball; and the pelvic floor muscle, which forms the base of the abdominal ball. It is important that all of these muscles contract together so that the increase in pressure is evenly distributed along the spine. This requires an element of control, which is sometimes lost through lack of practice. It therefore requires a conscious effort and a lot of practice to achieve this contraction of the inner unit.

NEED TO KNOW

Researchers have found that in people with chronic low back pain the inner unit muscles do not function correctly. Dysfunction of the inner unit could be one of the causes of low back pain.

THORACO-LUMBAR FASCIA GAIN

The *thoraco-lumbar fascia* is a sheet of connective tissue, almost tendon-like, that covers most of the muscles in the back and attaches to the spine, pelvis and sacrum. When the muscles of the inner unit are activated, tension is produced in the thoraco-lumbar fascia. It has been suggested that this tension creates an extension force on the spine (in other words, causes it to stiffen) and thus provides a degree of stabilisation that contributes to the overall stabilisation of the spine. The exact mechanism of thoraco-lumbar fascia gain is still under investigation and a topic of much debate.

HYDRAULIC AMPLIFIER EFFECT

When the erector spinae muscles contract, the thoraco-lumbar fascia that surrounds these muscles resists their expansion. This resistance increases the strength of the erector spinae muscles by up to 30 per cent, and therefore it can be assumed that this effect contributes in some way to the stabilisation of the spine. Again, like thoraco-lumbar fascia gain, the hydraulic amplifier effect is currently being researched and the exact mechanisms are not yet fully understood.

TASK

Briefly explain the mechanisms that contribute to the overall stabilisation of the spine.

Neutral position or zone

The concept of the neutral position of the spine can be explained by thinking about the gears in a car. When a car is in neutral, there is no torque, or turning force on the gearbox. However, when the gears are engaged, considerable force is applied to make the car move. Similarly, when a normal functional spine is in its *neutral zone* (also known as *neutral spine*), which is approximately midway between full posterior and anterior tilts of the pelvis, minimal force is placed on the spine and the structures that surround it (tendons, cartilage and ligaments). Any movement away from this position dramatically increases the stress placed on the surrounding tissues and hence the spine itself. Stabilisation control to maintain neutral spine is required when carrying out simple tasks such as sitting, as well as performing more complex tasks such as changing direction while running at speed, in order to prevent undue stress on the surrounding tissues that might eventually lead to injury. As mentioned before, this stabilisation control appears to be lacking in the majority of people who suffer from back pain and is thought to be one of the major causes of the back pain or injury responsible for the pain.

Awareness of the body and the position of its segments is a complex skill that requires practice – something that is made evident by the number of people who display poor posture. What appears to be neutral spine to an individual may not be considered neutral by the observer. Neutral spine can be found with the help of an observer by either standing or sitting on a stability ball and tilting the pelvis back and forward until the neutral position is found (see page 132). Tilting the pelvis forward (anterior tilt) increases the hollow in the lumbar spine area, whereas tilting the pelvis backwards (posterior tilt) flattens the lumbar spine area. This method of finding neutral spine is not an exact science, but can be used to help the general population gain an awareness of posture. Instructors should be aware that if an individual has difficulty in achieving neutral zone then they may need to be referred to a person qualified to make a postural assessment.

• Practitioner

1. Sit in an upright position on the stability ball with the knee joint just below the level of the hip joint and the feet shoulder-width apart.
2. Attempt to flatten the lower spine by pulling the crotch area up towards the chest (posterior tilt – see Exercise 1c).
3. Attempt to increase the hollow in the lower back by pulling the buttocks in a straight line towards the shoulder blades (anterior tilt – see Exercise 1a).
4. Repeat this movement several times at a slow, controlled pace.
5. Try to find the neutral position, after being informed of the correct position by the observer (see Exercise 1b).

• Observer

1. Make sure that any movement occurs only in the lumbar spine; do not allow any movement at the shoulders or in the legs.
2. Watch for the full range of motion between the full anterior and the full posterior tilt. Inform the practitioner when the pelvis is midway between these two points.

• Practitioner

1. Stand in an upright position with the feet shoulder-width apart.
2. Attempt to flatten the lower spine by pulling the crotch area up towards the chest. (See Exercise 2a).
3. Attempt to increase the hollow in the lower back by pulling the buttocks in a straight line towards the shoulder blades. (See Exercise 2b).
4. Repeat this movement several times at a slow, controlled pace.
5. Try to find the neutral position after being informed of the correct position by the observer. (See Exercise 2c).

EXERCISE 1 (A–C)

Seated procedure for finding the neutral spine

• Observer

1. Make sure that any movement occurs only in the lumbar spine; do not allow any movement at the shoulders or in the legs.
2. Watch for the full range of motion between the full anterior and the full posterior tilt.
3. Inform the practitioner when the pelvis is midway between these two points.

NEED TO KNOW

To help prevent any unwanted movement, the observer can place both hands on the shoulders of the practitioner. The observer will feel any unwanted movement.

Contraction of the transversus abdominis (TA)

One of the mechanisms that can be used to achieve stabilisation of the spine is the principle known as the abdominal or *fluid ball* technique, as described on page 130. Through the contraction of certain stabilising muscles, pressure is placed upon the spine, which prevents unwanted movement and helps the spine to work as a unit. It would be almost impossible to consciously contract all of the muscles associated with stabilisation. When the transversus abdominis muscle is contracted either consciously or sub-consciously, the other muscles of the inner unit contract immediately afterwards.

EXERCISE 2 (A–C)

Standing procedure for finding the neutral spine

Contraction of the stabilising muscles (inner unit) can be very difficult for several reasons. Many years of misuse, poor posture, overuse and weakness can result in a lack of subconscious activation of these muscles. As a result, it is common for exercises to be taught that are designed to improve subconscious activation of the inner unit muscles. One of the main difficulties associated with conscious activation is that many individuals try too hard, which usually results in the holding of breath and an increase in blood pressure. Research has suggested that only 30 per cent of the maximum contraction capability of the inner unit muscles is needed to create sufficient intra-abdominal pressure to stabilise the spine (Richardson et al., 2003).

Contraction of the transversus abdominis can be one of the most difficult conscious tasks for an individual to perform. However, for the contraction of the stabilising muscles to become subconscious (autonomous), it is essential to perform conscious practice of muscle contraction on a regular basis. The following method may be used to practise contraction of the transversus muscle, which will in turn activate the other stabilising muscles.

CONSCIOUS ACTIVATION OF THE TRANSVERSUS ABDOMINIS

• **Body position** Lie with your back on the floor, knees bent and feet flat on the floor. Relax and try not to flatten the spine against the floor; instead, maintain a normal lumbar curve.

• **Hand position** Find a position two inches below the navel and two inches to either side of that position. Press in lightly on each side using the first two fingers of each hand. This should be

133

the location of the transversus abdominis. Slide one hand under the natural curve of the lower spine so that you can feel any pressure changes from the body through the hand.

● **Initial contraction**   Cough! As the transversus abdominis is one of the muscles responsible for the forced expiration of air during coughing, you should feel the contraction under your fingers (that is, you should feel the muscle getting harder). The pressure on the hand under the lumbar spine should not change. Try to maintain constant pressure throughout the contraction.

● **Practice**   The aim of the exercise is to try to replicate the contraction felt when coughing, without actually coughing. This can sometimes take a considerable amount of time to achieve, but once you can do it aim to contract at about 30 per cent of your maximum contraction capability.

● **Progression**   Once you can contract the transversus abdominis, perform the same action without holding your breath or activating the rectus abdominis (a common mistake found in most people). You can place a hand just below the diaphragm to check for contraction of the rectus abdominis.

The lying method of contraction is suitable for initial purposes. Once individuals are capable of contracting their transversus abdominis, use the same method in a standing position. This makes it easier for individuals to perform the exercise on a daily basis.

The length of time, number of repetitions and frequency of practice of conscious contraction required to develop subconscious contraction control is different for every individual. It can be a lengthy process lasting up to several months, so it is recommended that conscious contraction practice be maintained for a period of no less than six months.

Typical core stability exercises

Once individuals are capable of contracting the transversus abdominis by conscious control, they can progress to other types of common stabilisation exercises. Individuals with no history of performing stabilisation exercises should initially be prescribed the most basic exercises and should only progress to more difficult exercises when they are comfortable with the previous level of stabilisation exercise.

The following core stability exercises should not be prescribed to clients who have back problems or who report pain when performing the exercises. Simple screening procedures (see chapter 11) should be sufficient to identify individuals who should not be prescribed stabilisation exercises. The exercises might need to be deferred until the individual has been referred to a relevant professional and has been authorised to carry out an exercise programme.

FLOOR EXERCISES

EXERCISE 3

Kneeling abdominal hollow

• Starting position

1. Kneel on the floor with your shoulders directly above your hands and your hips directly above your knees.
2. Keep your head facing down towards the floor to prevent undue stress on the cervical spine.
3. Keep your knees shoulder-width apart. Check that your spine is in the neutral position.

• Action

1. Consciously contract your transversus abdominis.
2. Breathe gently in and out, maintaining the contraction.
3. Breathe out and, before breathing in again, try to hollow your lower abdominals (imagine pulling your navel towards your spine).

4. Continuing to breathe normally. Hold this position for a few seconds or until you are unable to hold it any more.
5. Repeat, trying to maintain normal breathing throughout.
6. Concentrate on maintaining the starting position during the course of the exercise.

• Progressions

1. Try to perform the action without contracting the rectus abdominis.
2. Once you are comfortable with performing abdominal hollowing on all fours, try to perform the action in a standing position.
3. Try to contract the transversus abdominis without drawing in the lower abdominals. This is known as *abdominal bracing*.

EXERCISE 4

(a) and (b) Supine foot slide

• Starting position

1. Lie on your back with your feet flat on the floor and your knees bent as much as is comfortably possible.
2. Place one arm down by your side and the other under the lumbar spine to check the pressure on your hand throughout the exercise.
3. Keep your knees shoulder-width apart. Check that your spine is in the neutral position.

• Action

1. Consciously contract your transversus abdominis.
2. Breathe gently in and out.
3. Slowly slide one foot outwards along the floor until your leg is fully extended.

4. Return to the start position, trying to maintain normal breathing throughout.
5. Concentrate on keeping your spine in the neutral position during the exercise so that the pressure on your hand does not change.

• Progressions

1. Once you are comfortable with the above action, try increasing the speed of the movement slightly.
2. Once you can perform the above exercise without a change in pressure on the hand under the lumbar spine, try sliding both legs out and back at the same time.

EXERCISE 5

(a) and (b) Pelvic tilts

• Starting position

1. Lie on your back with your feet flat on the floor and your knees bent as much as is comfortably possible.
2. Place your arms by your sides or across your abdomen.
3. Keep your knees shoulder-width apart. Check that your spine is in the neutral position.

• Action

1. Consciously contract your transversus abdominis.
2. Breathe in and out gently.
3. Tilt your pelvis backward so that your lower back is flat on the floor (see Exercise 5b).
4. Return to the starting position, trying to maintain normal breathing throughout.

• Progressions

1. Try performing the exercise while lifting one foot slightly off the floor.
2. As well as tilting the pelvis backward, try to tilt it forward so that your lumbar spine is more arched than normal.

EXERCISE 6

(a) and (b) Side bridge

• Starting position

1. Lie on your side with your feet slightly apart to create a stable base.
2. Bend the arm nearest the floor at the elbow and rest it on the floor. This will provide support when you lift your upper body off the floor.
3. Put the opposite arm down by your side. Check that your spine is in the neutral position.
4. Keep your upper hip in line with your lower hip (see Exercise 6a).

• Action

1. Consciously contract your transversus abdominis.
2. Breathe gently in and out.

3. Raise your lower hip off the floor so that your body forms a straight line (see Exercise 6b).
4. Hold this position until you start to feel muscle fatigue.
5. Try to maintain normal breathing throughout.
6. Concentrate on keeping your spine in the neutral position during the exercise.

• Progressions

Once you are comfortable with the above exercise, start with the hip in the raised position. Try to lower the hip nearest the floor towards the floor, then raise it to the start position again. Repeat.

EXERCISE 7

(a) and (b) Prone plank

• Starting position

1. Lie on your front with your feet slightly apart to create a stable base.
2. Place your forearms on the floor with your hands approximately at face level. This will provide support when you lift your body off the floor (see Exercise 7a).

• Action

1. Consciously contract your transversus abdominis.
2. Breathe gently in and out.

3. Raise your body off the floor so that your body forms a straight line (see Exercise 7b).
4. Hold this position until you start to feel muscle fatigue.
5. Try to maintain normal breathing throughout.
6. Concentrate on keeping your spine in the neutral position during the exercise.

• Progression

Once you are comfortable with the above exercise, try a plank position with straight arms.

EXERCISE 8

(a) and (b) Supine plank

- ## Starting position

1. Sit on the floor with knees slightly apart and hands resting on the floor by the sides.
2. Bend your knees to approximately 90 degrees and keep your feet flat on the floor and your arms by your side. This will provide support when you lift your body off the floor (see Exercise 8a).

- ## Action

1. Consciously contract your transversus abdominis.
2. Breathe gently in and out.

3. Raise your body off the floor so that your body forms a straight line (see Exercise 8b).
4. Hold this position until you start to feel muscle fatigue.
5. Try to maintain normal breathing throughout.
6. Concentrate on keeping your spine in the neutral position during the exercise.

- ## Progression

Once you are comfortable with the above exercise, try keeping the plank position but raise one leg straight out in front.

STABILITY BALL EXERCISES

EXERCISE 9

Shoulder bridge

• Starting position

1. Lie face up with the ball under your shoulder blades.
2. Rest your head back onto the ball.
3. Keep your feet shoulder-width apart and your arms outstretched with the palms facing down.
4. Check that your spine is in the neutral position.
5. Walk your feet forward and lean back at the same time until the ball is under your shoulder blades.
6. Keep a straight horizontal line through your shoulder, knee and hip joints.

• Action

1. Consciously contract your transversus abdominis.

2. With your feet shoulder-width apart and your arms outstretched, gently roll a few inches to one side at the shoulders, then return to the starting point.
3. Repeat, but roll to the opposite side.
4. Repeat this five times to each side.
5. Maintain normal breathing throughout.

• Safety point

Roll only as far as you feel in control of the movement. Use your hands to prevent yourself rolling if you go too far.

EXERCISE 10

Foot bridge

• Starting position

1. Lie face up on the floor
2. Place the soles of your feet midway between the top and the side of the ball. Your knee joints should be at about 90 degrees at this point.
3. Keep your feet shoulder-width apart and your arms outstretched on the floor.
4. Raise your bottom off the floor until your spine is in the neutral position. Your legs tend to straighten at this point.
5. Only your shoulder blades, head and arms should be resting on the floor.

• Action

1. Consciously contract your transversus abdominis.

2. With your feet shoulder-width apart and your arms outstretched, use your feet to roll the ball gently a few inches to one side, then return to the starting point.
3. Repeat, but roll to the opposite side.
4. Repeat five times to each side.
5. Maintain normal breathing throughout.
6. Concentrate on maintaining the starting position during the exercise.

• Safety point

Roll only as far as you feel in control of the movement. If you lose control, adopt the starting position and repeat from the point at which you lost control.

EXERCISE 11

Straight-leg bridge

● Starting position

1. Lie face up on the floor.
2. Place the ball under your feet just below your heels.
3. Keep your feet shoulder-width apart and your arms outstretched on the floor.
4. Raise your bottom off the floor until your spine is in the neutral position.
5. There should be a straight line through the knee and hip joint.
6. Only your shoulder blades, head and arms should be resting on the floor.

● Action

1. Consciously contract your transversus abdominis.

2. With your feet shoulder-width apart and your arms outstretched, use your feet to roll the ball gently a few inches to one side, then return to the starting point.
3. Repeat, but roll to the opposite side.
4. Repeat five times to each side.
5. Maintain normal breathing throughout.
6. Concentrate on maintaining the starting position during the exercise.

● Safety point

Roll only as far as you feel in control of the movement. If you lose control, adopt the starting position and repeat from the point at which you lost control.

EXERCISE 12

Front bridge

• Starting position

1. Kneel on the floor in front of the ball.
2. Lean forward over the ball so that your chest rests on the ball.
3. Roll over the top of the ball so that your forearms rest on the floor in front of the ball and your pelvis rests directly on top of the ball.
4. Check that your spine is in the neutral position.
5. Keep your neck in neutral by looking down at the floor.
6. Maintain a straight line through your knee, hip and shoulder joints.

• Action

1. Consciously contract your transversus abdominis.

2. With your feet together and your forearms on the floor, gently roll the ball a few inches to one side and then return to the starting point.
3. Repeat, but roll to the opposite side.
4. Repeat five times to each side.
5. Maintain normal breathing throughout.
6. Concentrate on maintaining the starting position during the exercise.

• Safety point

Roll only as far as you feel in control of the movement. Put one foot on the floor if you feel you are about to lose control.

EXERCISE 13

Ab burner

• Starting position

1. Kneel on the floor about 3 feet in front of the ball.
2. Lean forward over the ball so that your forearms rest on the ball.
3. Keep your knees shoulder-width apart.
4. Check that your spine is in the neutral position.
5. Keep your neck in neutral by looking at the floor in front of the ball.

• Action

1. Consciously contract your transversus abdominis.

2. With your knees shoulder-width apart and your forearms on the ball, gently roll the ball a few inches to one side and then return to the starting point.
3. Repeat, but roll to the opposite side.
4. Repeat five times to each side.
5. Maintain normal breathing throughout.
6. Concentrate on maintaining the starting position during the exercise.

• Safety point

Roll only as far as you feel in control of the movement. Use your hands to prevent yourself rolling if you go too far.

EXERCISE 14

(a) and (b) Floor push

 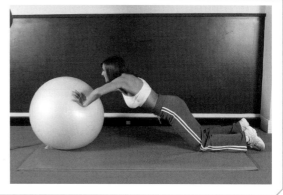

• Starting position

1. Kneel on the floor about 3 feet in front of the ball.
2. Lean forward over the ball so that your hands rest on the ball.
3. Keep your knees shoulder-width apart.
4. Check that your spine is in the neutral position.
5. Keep your neck in neutral by looking at the floor in front of the ball.

• Action

1. Consciously contract your transversus abdominis.

2. With the knees shoulder-width apart and your hands on the ball, gently lower your body until your chest comes to rest on the ball.
3. Gently raise your body back to the starting point by straightening your arms.
4. Repeat 10 times.
5. Maintain normal breathing throughout.
6. Concentrate on maintaining the starting position during the exercise.

• Safety point

Lower your body only as far as feels comfortable.

Exercise guidelines

FIG. 9.9

In all new fitness or health programmes there is a period known as *habituation* during which the body, in particular the brain, becomes accustomed to the new form of exercise. When the brain becomes accustomed to the exercise, the body will adapt physically in order to accommodate the new level of exercise placed upon it. This period may last for several months. At this stage, the level of exercise can either be increased or maintained, depending on the individual's goals. Many factors influence the speed at which the body becomes accustomed to the new exercise regime or programme, such as frequency, duration, number of repetitions and ability level.

Typical intervertebral disc pressures (kg/cm²)

FREQUENCY

Frequency is how often something occurs. In exercise, this is related to the number of times per week that the exercises are carried out. At the start of any new programme at least two sessions per week are recommended in order for the body to adapt to cope with the regularity of the routine. Once the exercises have been carried out regularly for a period of a few weeks, the frequency of sessions can be reduced to once a week in order to maintain the adaptations that the body has made.

DURATION

Duration relates to the amount of time spent on each exercise. The actual research carried out in this area is conflicting and there is no consensus as to the ideal duration of any one exercise. Every individual has a different objective and a different ability level, so it is impossible to recommend a duration period

that would benefit all individuals equally. As a general guide, however, start with an exercise duration of about 15 seconds. If the individual feels capable of increasing the duration, start by adding a period of five seconds to each exercise. If the individual feels that the duration for the exercise is too long, reduce the time of each exercise by five seconds until you reach a suitable duration.

NEED TO KNOW

Core stability training is effective when performed at a comfortable level; the 'no pain, no gain' saying is definitely not recommended in this case.

FIG. 9.10

A herniated (or slipped) disc

Spinal cord

Articulating process

Slipped disk

Nerve root

Vertebral body

REPETITIONS

The number of repetitions simply refers to the number of times the exercise is repeated without a break. As core stability is not a strength issue, but relates to a learning process of the brain, the focus is on repeating the exercises at regular intervals to achieve this learning process as quickly as possible. Again, as research is unclear on the ideal number of repetitions, adjust the number of repetitions of each exercise to suit each individual's ability level. Once an individual becomes comfortable with this number of repetitions and feels able to perform more, increase the number until you reach a comfortable level.

NEED TO KNOW

If time is a concern, attempt as many repetitions as you are able. The old saying applies: 'Anything is better than nothing'.

SPINAL COMPRESSION FORCES

Research has demonstrated that there are varying degrees of intervertebral disc compression forces, depending on the exercise that is performed or the position of the body. In relation to exercise, Fig. 9.9 shows intervertebral disc pressures in various positions, adapted from the *Journal of Spinal Research Foundation*.

When the spine is in neutral, as previously described, intervertebral discs are capable of withstanding large amounts of pressure as forces are evenly distributed. If the spine is not in neutral, however, there is a 'squeezing' effect of the intervertebral disc due to uneven pressure. This can result in a protrusion of the inner layer of the disc (nucleus pulposis) through the outer layer (annulus fibrosus), which is known as a disc herniation (or more commonly, a slipped disc). See Fig. 9.10.

EXAMPLE QUESTIONS

9.1 Which of the following properties relates to stabilising muscles?

a) short-term, explosive, phasic, fast-twitch

b) postural, endurance, phasic, fast-twitch

c) short-term, endurance, phasic, slow-twitch

d) postural, endurance, tonic, slow-twitch

9.2 Which of the following properties relates to mobilising muscles?

a) short-term, explosive, phasic, slow-twitch

b) postural, endurance, phasic, fast-twitch

c) short-term, explosive, phasic, fast-twitch

d) postural, endurance, tonic, slow-twitch

9.3 Which of the following can be considered to be predominantly stabilising muscles for the core?

a) internal oblique, rectus abdominis, diaphragm

b) multifidus, transversus abdominis, pelvic floor

c) pelvic floor, external oblique, diaphragm

d) multifidus, erector spinae, internal oblique

9.4 Which of the following can be considered to be predominantly mobilising muscles for the core?

a) internal oblique, rectus abdominis, diaphragm

b) multifidus, transversus abdominis, pelvic floor

c) erector spinae, external oblique, rectus abdominis

d) multifidus, erector spinae, internal oblique

9.5 Which of the following can be considered to be a predominantly stabilising muscle for the hip joint?

a) internal obliques

b) gluteus maximus

c) transversus abdominis

d) gluteus medius

9.6 Which of the following can be considered to be predominantly a mobilising muscle for the hip joint?

a) internal obliques

b) gluteus maximus

    c) transversus abdominis

    d) gluteus medius

9.7 When local muscles contract to compress the 'fluid ball' in the abdomen it is known as what?

    a) neutral spine or zone

    b) intra-abdominal pressure

    c) hydraulic amplifier effect

    d) thoraco-lumbar fascia gain

9.8 An increase in the tension of the connective tissues in the spinal region is known as what?

    a) neutral spine or zone

    b) intra-abdominal pressure

    c) fluid ball pressure

    d) thoraco-lumbar fascia gain

9.9 Research has suggested that what percentage of maximum contraction is sufficient to create sufficient intra-abdominal pressure to stabilise the spine?

    a) 70

    b) 100

    c) 50

    d) 30

9.10 What best relates to the statement *'when there is minimal force placed on the spine and the structures that surround it such as tendons, cartilage and ligaments'*?

    a) anterior pelvic tilt

    b) neutral zone

    c) intra-abdominal pressure

    d) thoraco-lumbar fascia gain

9.11 True or false? Normal screening procedures should be carried out prior to prescribing core stabilisation exercises but those with back problems should be excluded.

    True   False

9.12 The length of time, number of repetitions and frequency of practice of conscious contraction required to develop subconscious contraction control of the transversus abdominis can take up to how long?

    a) a few hours

    b) a few days

    c) a few weeks

    d) a few months

Further reading

Abrahams, P., Craven, J. and Lumley, J. (2011) *Illustrated Clinical Anatomy* (2nd ed.), Hodder Arnold

Handzel, T.M. (2003) 'Core training for improved performance', *NSCA's Performance Training Journal*, 2(6): 26–30

Liddle, D.S., Baxterb, D.G. and Graceya, J.H. (2009) 'Physiotherapists' use of advice and exercise for the management of chronic low back pain: A national survey', *Manual Therapy*, 14(2): 189–196

Marshall, P.W. and Murphy, B.A. (2005) 'Core stability exercises on and off a Swiss ball', *Archives of Physical Medicine and Rehabilitation*, 86(2): 242–249

Norris, C.M. (2009) *The Complete Guide to Abdominal Training*, Bloomsbury

Norris, C.M. (2001) *Back Stability* (2nd ed.), Human Kinetics

Porter, S. (2008) *The Anatomy Workbook* (2nd ed.), Butterworth Heinemann

Richardson, C., Jull, G., Hodges, P. and Hides, J. (2003) *Therapeutic Exercise for Spinal Segmental Stabilization in Low Back Pain*, Churchill Livingstone

Ross, J.S. and Wilson, J.W. (2018) *Anatomy and Physiology in Health and Illness* (13th ed.), Churchill Livingstone

Sewell, D., Watkins, P. and Griffin, M. (2012) *Sport and Exercise Science: An Introduction* (2nd ed.), Hodder Arnold

Tortora, G.J. and Grabowski, S.R. (2017) *Principles of Anatomy and Physiology* (15th ed.), Wiley

Components and Principles of Fitness

10

OBJECTIVES

After completing this chapter, you will be able to:

1 Define the terms 'physical fitness', 'wellness' and 'health-related fitness'.
2 Define the term 'hypokinetic disease'.
3 List and describe the components of fitness.
4 State the ACSM guidelines relating to the components of fitness.
5 Describe how components of fitness can affect the body.
6 Explain the factors affecting physical fitness.
7 List and describe the principles of fitness.
8 List the main health risks associated with inactivity.

Introduction

This chapter deals with the components and principles of fitness in relation to guidelines within the Professional Standards framework for health and fitness, within which instructors should be able to identify the components and principles of fitness and list the guidelines associated with these.

Later chapters in the book provide information regarding the practical application of theoretical knowledge, which, along with the content covered in this chapter, will provide you with the understanding and ability to design appropriate exercise programmes for apparently healthy individuals in line with current guidelines for exercise.

Definitions of fitness

There are many definitions and individual perceptions of 'fitness'. For some, fitness might include the ability to perform some activity at a competitive level, while to others it might be the ability to perform everyday tasks without undue stress and fatigue. Fitness might also include a health or wellness component, which can relate to the absence of disease.

HEALTH-RELATED PHYSICAL FITNESS

The American College of Sports Medicine (ACSM) defines health-related physical fitness as 'an ability to perform daily activities with vigour and the demonstration of traits and capacities that are associated with a low risk of premature development of hypokinetic diseases'.

The closest translation for the word *hypokinetic* is 'low movement'. Hypokinetic diseases are associated with low levels of activity, such as heart disease, obesity and high blood pressure. For the purpose of this book, it is assumed that any prescribed exercise, regardless of the definition of fitness, will be beneficial in reducing the risk of hypokinetic disease.

WELLNESS

The ACSM definition of health-related physical fitness relates only to physical well-being, not to psychological well-being. However, there are many advocates of the notion that exercise can have a positive psychological effect – for example, promoting mental, social and emotional well-being. The World Health Organization (WHO) promotes the idea of *wellness*, defining it as 'a state of complete physical, mental and social well-being, and not merely the absence of disease or infirmity'.

PHYSICAL FITNESS

Although the terms health-related physical fitness and wellness can be defined clearly, the most common anecdotal term used within the health and fitness industry is *fitness*. The ACSM distinguishes between health-related physical fitness and physical fitness, defining the latter as 'a set of attributes that relates to the ability to perform physical activity'.

Components of physical fitness

Fitness, or to be more precise, physical fitness, can be divided into discrete components that can be trained or adapted individually. Depending on the type of training carried out, an individual can be classed as 'fit' in one or more of the individual components.

The ACSM lists the following components of health-related physical fitness: *cardiovascular endurance, muscular strength, muscular endurance, body composition* and *flexibility*. The components of physical fitness are the same, but also include *motor skills*, which comprise several sub-components. This book focuses on the components of health-related physical fitness.

CARDIOVASCULAR ENDURANCE

Cardiovascular endurance is the ability of the heart and lungs to deliver oxygen to the working muscles (sometimes known as *aerobic capacity*) and for the muscles to use this oxygen to generate work.

● **Measuring cardiovascular endurance** Cardiovascular endurance can be measured as *volume of oxygen* (VO_2). As the exercise intensity increases, the volume of oxygen consumed increases directly until it reaches a plateau, as shown in Fig. 10.1. This plateau is

FIG. 10.1

Relationship between exercise intensity and volume of oxygen

termed 'VO$_2$ max' and is also commonly known as 'aerobic capacity', 'aerobic power' or 'maximal oxygen uptake'. The units used to measure VO$_2$ are millilitres of oxygen per kilogram bodyweight per minute (mlO$_2$.kg^{-1}min^{-1}).

Testing can be done either at sub-maximal levels or at maximum capability depending on the experience of the individual being tested, the experience of the tester and the goal of the test. Testing to maximum levels or capability is referred to as a VO$_2$ max test. Some of the common methods of testing for VO$_2$ include the Conconi test, Cooper Test, Balke Test, Multi-stage Fitness Test (also known as the Beep Test) and the Rockport Walking Test. Fig. 10.2 shows typical VO$_2$ levels that can be achieved.

• How to improve cardiovascular endurance
The best types of exercise for improving cardiovascular endurance are those that involve the use of large muscle groups over a prolonged period of time at an intensity that is classed as aerobic (for example, walking, hiking, running, stepping, swimming, cycling, dancing,

skiing, skipping and so on). As the intensity of the exercise increases, the amount of oxygen required to cope with the demands made by the muscles increases; therefore, the heart rate increases in proportion. This increase in heart rate due to an increase in exercise intensity is known as a *linear relationship*. In other words, there is an equal increase in heart rate for an equal increase in intensity. Fig. 10.3 shows that after performing regular cardiovascular exercise for a period of time, the same intensity (speed) can usually be maintained with a lower heart rate.

• FITT guidelines for cardiovascular training
It can be difficult to know the correct duration and intensity of exercise to recommend in order for clients to achieve optimum benefits in terms of cardiovascular endurance.

Too little exercise might not have the desired effect, whereas too much might result in a condition known as *over-training*, where damage to the body may occur in the form of an injury or a respiratory disease such as the common

FIG. 10.2

Typical VO$_2$ levels

FIG. 10.3

Heart rate against speed for pre- and post-training

TABLE 10.1

FITT guidelines for cardiovascular training	
Frequency	**Three–five days per week >3 days vigorous, >5 days moderate**
Intensity	55–90% of maximum heart rate (RPE 12–16: see page 256)
Time	30–60 minutes moderate aerobic exercise or 20–60 minutes vigorous
Type	Regular major muscle groups

cold. For this reason, the ACSM has developed guidelines known as the *FITT principles*, which are recommended by governing bodies across Europe. FITT stands for *frequency, intensity, time* and *type*. Table 10.1 outlines the FITT guidelines for cardiovascular training.

Some clients may not be able to achieve 20 minutes of cardiovascular exercise or maintain intensities above 55 per cent of maximum heart rate. Therefore, the guidelines should be used to set targets for clients, rather than being absolute goals that clients must achieve. Any progressions should be limited to an increase of no more than 20 per cent of duration each week until clients can exercise at a moderate to vigorous intensity for 20–60 minutes. Increases in duration and frequency usually precede intensity increases.

● **Benefits of cardiovascular endurance** There are many benefits associated with an increase in cardiovascular endurance. One of the most important is a reduced risk in Coronary Artery Disease (CAD), and other benefits include:

- reduced blood pressure
- reduced body fat
- lower heart rate for given intensity of exercise
- increased exercise threshold for accumulation of blood lactate (the performer can exercise at a higher intensity before lactic acid builds up to the point at which intensity has to be reduced)
- increase in HDL (good) cholesterol

MUSCULAR STRENGTH

Muscular strength is the maximum amount of force that a muscle or muscle group can generate.

● **Measuring muscular strength** Both static and dynamic muscular strength can be measured. In static strength testing, machines called dynamometers measure how much force an individual can exert against it without any movement. In dynamic strength testing, an individual moves an external load (usually free weights or resistance machines). This is known as *1 repetition maximum* testing or *1RM* testing, where the maximum amount of weight that can be lifted once with good form is recorded. It is possible to predict 1RM from multiple RM testing; for example, 6RM is the maximum amount of weight that can be lifted six times, which can then be used to predict 1RM.

● **How to improve muscular strength** Muscular strength can be developed through resistance training, including using machine and free weights, bodyweight and resistance bands. Developing muscular strength normally requires relatively high resistance (or weight) and few repetitions, and is usually associated with an increase in muscle size. Because of the intense nature of this type of training, it is common for individuals to experience pain or stiffness in the muscles that have been trained in the days following a training session. This sensation is known as delayed onset muscle soreness or DOMS.

MUSCULAR ENDURANCE

Muscular endurance is the ability of a muscle or muscle group to perform repeated contractions against a resistance over a period of time, and is associated with resistance training using relatively low intensity and high repetitions. Hypertrophy is not usually associated with this type of training, although DOMS can be experienced if training is carried out to fatigue. Testing normally involves recording the maximum number of repetitions of a task, such as a push-up or sit-up that can be achieved.

• **Benefits of resistance training** There are many benefits of resistance training that vary slightly depending on the type of training. The benefits include the following:

• increase in muscle mass, which increases resting metabolic rate

• increase in bone mass
• reduced risk of osteoporosis
• increased glucose tolerance
• increase in joint integrity
• improved posture
• reduction in back pain
• reduced risk of hypertension
• reduced risk of diabetes

The benefits of muscular endurance training are similar to those of muscular strength training, but with less emphasis on increased muscle mass and more emphasis on muscle tone. One of the long-term effects of resistance training is hypertrophy, or an increase in the size of the muscle being trained. This usually occurs after the first few weeks of training, as strength gains in the first few weeks are as a result of 'learning' mechanisms known as *neural* changes.

Delayed-onset muscle soreness (DOMS) can occur a day or two after a particularly intense training session. Light aerobic exercise following resistance training can reduce this effect.

• **FITT guidelines for resistance training** Table 10.2 outlines the FITT guidelines for resistance training.

Note: ACSM guidelines recommend a timing sequence of three seconds concentric and three seconds eccentric contraction for all resistance exercises that involve a full range of motion.

TABLE 10.2

FITT principles for resistance training	
Frequency	2–3 non-consecutive sessions per week each major muscle group
Intensity	Novice 60–70% of IRM, experienced ≥80% of IRM
Time	Strength/power 8–12 RM. Endurance 15 RM. 2–4 sets
Type	Major agonist/antagonist pairs

Volitional fatigue is the point at which the individual performing the exercise thinks that he or she can no longer carry on. This can be uncomfortable for the performer, so to encourage adherence to an exercise programme it is sensible to adopt a flexible approach to this guideline for individuals who are not familiar with exercising to fatigue levels.

FLEXIBILITY

Flexibility is the ability to move a joint through its complete range of motion.

- **Testing flexibility** Flexibility is joint specific in that an individual may be flexible in one joint and not in another. Therefore, there is no one test that is whole-body specific and all joints must be assessed individually using *goniometry*, where the angle of each joint is measured and compared against tables for normal ranges of motion. A common flexibility test used in the health and fitness industry is the 'sit and reach' test, where an individual sits with straight legs and reaches forward to record the distance reached with the fingertips. This measures only hamstring and upper back flexibility.

- **Benefits of flexibility** One of the main benefits of maintaining the range of motion within joints is that it allows individuals to carry out daily activities as long as possible throughout their lives. Although it is frequently recommended that stretching can help prevent injury, there is little evidence to support the notion: it has been shown that a high degree as well as a low degree of flexibility can increase injury risk. It is recommended that people with tight muscles would probably benefit most from static stretching whereas those who are naturally supple should not engage in more than light stretching. The most effective stretching occurs when the muscles are warm.

- **Types of stretching** There are many types of stretching exercises, including *static*, *dynamic*, *PNF* and *ballistic*. Below is a simple description of the common types of stretches.

Static stretching

A static stretch is held for a period of time at a point of mild tension. The point of tension is usually the point at which the stretch reflex is invoked. If the stretch is held for long enough, the tension usually subsides and the stretch can be taken further, if required. If a partner or another group of muscles assists in the stretching process, it is known as an *active* stretch. If there is no assistance, it is a *passive* stretch. Research on the optimum time period for a stretch is vague, but guidelines relating to the recommended time period are shown in Table 10.3.

TABLE 10.3

FITT guidelines for flexibility training	
Frequency	Minimum 2–3 sessions per week; ideally 5–7 sessions per week
Intensity	To the end range of motion at a point of tightness, without pain
Time	10–30 seconds, 2–4 times per stretch
Type	Static, preceded by a warm-up

Dynamic stretching

A dynamic stretch refers to stretching in motion, where an agonist muscle is contracted to stretch an antagonist muscle. When this occurs it is known as reciprocal inhibition. This type of stretching is usually carried out in a slow and controlled manner in order to minimise the risk of injury and to mimic the types of movement that may be used in the exercises to follow.

Ballistic stretching

Ballistic stretches are bouncing movements caused by momentum or gravity. This type of stretching is usually carried out only by athletes who are familiar with this type of stretching: as there is little control of the movement, there is a greater risk of injury than with other types of stretching.

PNF stretching

PNF stands for proprioceptive neuromuscular facilitation. This is a type of partner-assisted stretching that is normally used for tight or injured muscles. With this type of stretch tension is built up in a muscle prior to it being stretched. When tension in a muscle reaches a certain level, the Golgi tendon organ (GTO) located at the musculo-tendonous junction causes a reflexive relaxation of the muscle during the subsequent stretch. This type of stretching requires training, so should be performed only by those who are qualified to do so. CRAC (Contraction Relax Antagonist Contract) is another form of this type of stretching.

Table 10.3 outlines the FITT guidelines for flexibility training.

BODY COMPOSITION

Body composition refers to the ratio of fat to lean tissue in an individual: in other words, how lean, overweight or obese a person is. Even though body composition is listed as a component of fitness, it is probably more accurate to associate it with an indication of health, as excess body fat is associated with hypertension, diabetes, stroke, coronary heart disease and hyperlipidaemia.

Body composition is also affected greatly by other components of fitness, such as cardiovascular and resistance training.

• Measuring body composition

Body composition can be measured in many different ways, including BMI, using skinfolds, underwater weighing and electrical impedance methods. Some methods are more accurate than others. One of the easiest methods is BMI, or body mass index. Although this is not a direct measurement of body fat percentage, it does give an indication of overweight or obesity, which has been defined by the ACSM as the percentage of body fat at which an individual's risk of disease increases. BMI is calculated using the following equation:

BMI=Weight (kg)/Height^2 (m^2)

Table 10.4 shows how BMI is used to classify body composition.

Although the causes of obesity can include hypothalmic, endocrine and genetic disorders, diet and physical inactivity are the prime factors. It is generally accepted and recommended by the ACSM that an increase in calorie expenditure and a decrease in calorie intake is the most effective long-term method

TABLE 10.4

BMI classifications	
BMI	**Classification**
<25	Normal
25–30	Overweight
>30	Obese

for treating obesity: between 150 and 400 kcal of daily energy expenditure is recommended for weight-loss programmes.

MOTOR SKILLS

Many sub-components are associated with motor skills, including speed, power, agility, coordination and balance. All of these areas can be improved with training.

• **Speed** Speed is the ability to move quickly from one point to another and can be improved through muscle coordination, efficient body movement, core strength and flexibility.

• **Power** Power is a combination of strength and speed and can be developed through plyometric and resistance training.

• **Agility** Agility is the ability to change direction at speed.

• **Balance** Balance is the ability to maintain equilibrium at all times. Proprioceptors in the body give information to the brain on the position of all limbs, as well as balance information from the inner ear and the eyes.

• **Coordination** Coordination is the ability to move the limbs precisely in a particular direction.
There are many theories regarding the storage of movement patterns, known as motor programmes. One theory proposed by Schmidt (1992) suggests that typical movements such as bending and squatting are stored with related information such as muscle timing and velocities. All other movements are just adaptations of these typical stored movements. For example, the movement sequence for a jump is similar to that of a squat because of the relationship of the body segments. A jump sequence, however, is entirely different from that of a leg press or leg extension. There are

no recommended guidelines for motor skills in relation to FITT principles.

TASK

List and briefly describe the components of fitness and state the recommended guidelines related to each component.

Factors influencing physical fitness

When training for any of the components of fitness, various factors may influence the outcome of the type of training. These factors include *body type*, *gender*, *fitness level*, *lifestyle* and *age*.

BODY TYPE

The distribution of fibre type within muscles is determined at birth. A person with a higher percentage distribution of fast-twitch fibres will be more predisposed to strength-type events, whereas a person with a high percentage of slow-twitch fibres will be predisposed to endurance-type events.

There are three extreme classifications of body type that can be used to describe the overall shape of an individual: *endomorph*, *ectomorph* and *mesomorph* (see Table 10.5). It is common for individuals to be a combination of more than one type, so a grading system for each classification can be used.

GENDER

Gender relates simply to either male or female. This has some implications on the components of fitness. For example, cardiovascular potential

TABLE 10.5

Characteristics of different body types	
Endomorph	A pear-shaped body A rounded head Wide hips and shoulders Wider front to back rather than side to side A lot of fat on the body, upper arms and thighs
Ectomorph	A high forehead A receding chin Narrow shoulders and hips A narrow chest and abdomen Thin arms and legs Little muscle and fat
Mesomorph	A wedge-shaped body A cubical head Wide, broad shoulders Muscled arms and legs Narrow hips Narrow from front to back rather than side to side

(VO$_2$ max) is typically 15–30 per cent lower in females than in males. Men are also capable of greater muscle hypertrophy as a result of strength training, as they tend to have a greater proportion of fast-twitch fibres.

FITNESS

A less fit individual will initially make greater improvements in components of fitness than a fitter person. This should be taken into account when setting goals and targets with clients (see chapter 12).

LIFESTYLE

There are many aspects of lifestyle that can affect components of fitness. One of the main aspects is psychological stress, which can

have a detrimental effect on the way in which individuals train. Smoking and drinking alcohol can have a similar effect.

AGE

Ageing can decrease the individual components of fitness, but with a regular training routine these diminishing effects can be minimised and in some cases reversed. For example, flexibility can very quickly be lost, but many older individuals retain flexibility by participating in exercises such as yoga.

TASK
Describe how various factors can influence physical fitness.

Principles of fitness

When designing any exercise programme it is important to remember certain fundamental factors that can have an effect on the outcome of the programme. These factors are called *principles of fitness*. These principles must be taken into account with all individuals in relation to the design of a training or exercise programme.

SPECIFICITY

The body can adapt to the demands of various types of exercise, and the type of adaptation that takes place is dependent on the muscle fibres involved and the types of exercise. For example, type 1 fibres will adapt to endurance training, while type 2 fibres will adapt to more intense strength training. The body will also adapt to the type (or specificity) of the training. For example, an individual who trains predominantly on a treadmill will become better at using the treadmill even though there will be a transfer of fitness to other types of cardio exercise.

ADAPTATION

This principle states that the adaptations derived from an exercise are specific to the exercise and to the muscles involved in that exercise. For example, runners show little improvement in the muscular endurance of their arm muscles, while cyclists show most of their muscular endurance improvement in their leg muscles. In order for adaptation in the body to occur, however, the body must be subjected to the exercise on a regular basis.

OVERLOAD

In order for an individual to adapt to a new demand or routine, overload must be achieved.

Overload can be described as 'taking the body or system to a point just beyond what it is usually accustomed to' (ACSM, 2018). If any system within the body (a muscle or an organ) is made to work harder than it normally does on a regular basis, it will undergo certain physical changes to adapt to the new workload. It is important to remember that the body should be taken to a workload just beyond normal levels; if it is taken too far, injury may occur. There are many ways in which overload can be achieved within a programme in order to achieve adaptation. Lever length, speed, resistance and gravity are among many variables in which to progress a programme of exercise.

- **Lever length** Increasing the length of the lever will increase the intensity of the exercise. For example, a straight-arm lateral raise will be made slightly easier by bending the elbows (bringing the weight closer to the body).

- **Speed** Slowing down the speed of movement will increase the intensity. Try doing a very slow resistance exercise with your usual weight.

- **Resistance** Increasing the resistance will obviously increase the intensity. Weights should be progressed when you are able to exceed the number of repetitions that was originally specified (see repetition maximum in chapter 14).

- **Gravity** The general principle is that when doing free-weight or body-weight exercise, the movement should be vertical (against gravity) to achieve the maximum intensity.

PROGRESSION

If the workload of a training programme is not progressed, the individual will not continue to adapt. Instead, once the body has adapted to the current workload, it will not attempt to adapt any further. In order to progress, the workload must be periodically changed once the body has become accustomed to the previous workload. The rate of progression is specific to each individual and can also be affected by various factors:

- **Fitness level** Less fit individuals will progress at a faster rate than fitter individuals.

- **Experience** An individual with past experience of certain exercises will progress at a faster rate than those with no experience.

- **Injury** An injury to a specific site can reverse any gains previously made at that site. It is important to remember that the rest of the body may be trained to prevent total body reversibility.

- **Environment** The nature of the environment can affect progression in several ways. For example, altitude training can have an effect on oxygen transport, while heat and cold can affect the rate of progression.

REGRESSION (REVERSIBILITY)

Just as the body can become stronger if the workload is increased, the body can also become weaker over a period of time if the workload is reduced. It is possible for specific fitness components to diminish within two weeks of cessation of exercise. This principle is known as *regression*.

INDIVIDUALITY

As all individuals progress at different rates, it is important that frequency, intensity and duration of exercise are manipulated to suit the individual. In any health-related fitness programme, individuals should be encouraged

to start slowly and begin at levels that can easily be maintained. Progression should then be encouraged when the individual feels that he or she can cope with the current workload and is able to progress.

RECOVERY TIME

It is often the case that the one thing missing from a progressive training programme is that of recovery time. It is obvious that rest is just as important in any exercise programme as active recovery periods. Instructors should constantly monitor individuals for signs of exhaustion and over-training, such as a drop in performance, increase in resting heart rate and regular illness. Recovery of the muscular, cardiovascular and neural systems depends on many factors, such as the intensity of the training session, individual fitness levels, age, psychological factors and dietary interventions. As a very general guideline, individuals should be given a 24–48-hour recovery period following a bout of exercise. This can be split, however, so that training can take place each day. With resistance training, for example, daily sessions could take place but different muscle groups could be targeted on different days to allow recovery.

TASK
List and briefly explain the principles used in prescribing exercise.

Health risks of inactivity

The benefits of undertaking regular physical activity are well documented throughout

TABLE 10.6

Health risks of inactivity

Condition	Incidence and effect of physical activity (PA)
Coronary heart disease (CHD)	In the UK about 38% of CHD related deaths are as a result of PA or sedentary lifestyles. Inactive people are almost twice as likely to have a heart attack as active people (Department of Health, 2000).
Stroke	According to the British Heart Foundation (2005), stroke accounts for about 9% of all deaths in men and about 13% of all deaths in women in the UK. Research suggests that moderately active people are less likely to have a stroke or die of stroke-related causes than those with low activity levels.
Certain cancers	It is estimated that more than 7,000 women in England alone died prematurely from breast cancer in the year 2000. It has been widely reported that regular PA is associated with a decreased risk of developing colon cancer by up to 50%. Although it would be difficult to measure the positive impact on these figures it is recommended that sedentary females should become more active.
Diabetes	About 1.5 million people in the UK have been diagnosed with Type 2 diabetes. Regular PA can lower the risk of developing non-insulin dependent diabetes mellitus by as much as 50% (NHS, 2009).
Hypertension	High blood pressure affects more than 16 million people in the UK and is the direct cause of about half of all strokes and heart attacks in the country. Regular PA prevents or delays the development of high blood pressure (Health Survey for England, 2007).
Osteoporosis	According to Van Staa (2001), in the UK about 1 in 2 women and 1 in 5 men over the age of 50 will sustain a spine, hip or wrist fracture mainly as a result of osteoporosis. Strength training in older women has been shown to reduce the risk of hip fracture by up to 50%.
Obesity	In England, in 2007, about 65% of men and 56% of women were overweight (this is including those that are obese). Regular PA can reduce the risk of becoming obese by as much as 50% compared to people with sedentary lifestyles (NHS, 2009)
Anxiety and depression	Regular PA appears to relieve symptoms of depression and anxiety, improve mood and self-esteem, and protect against the development of mild forms of depression (Kugler, 1994 and Boutcher, 2000)
Osteoarthritis	According to the Arthritis Research Campaign in 2002, arthritis (in all forms) affects about 7 million people (more than 10%) in the UK at any one time. Research has shown that an absence of stress on the joints can increase the risk of osteoarthritis (as can an excess of stress)

this book. However, it should be noted that there are many health risks associated with inactivity. In 2002, a report from the World Health Organization (WHO) stated that physical inactivity (less than 2.5 hours per week moderate intensity activity or 1 hour per week of vigorous activity) is one of the ten leading causes of death in developed countries, resulting in more than 1.9 million deaths worldwide per year. There are many published reports that discuss the range of health risks associated with physical inactivity (or being sedentary, as it is usually referred to) of which Table 10.6 shows common examples. For information purposes, the Department of Health (2004) classified active people as having an energy expenditure of 500–1,000 kcals per week, which is about 6 to 12 miles of walking (roughly 10,000 to 20,000 steps per week) for an average-weight individual.

EXAMPLE QUESTIONS

10.1 The ACSM defines what as *'an ability to perform daily activities with vigour and the demonstration of traits and capacities that are associated with a low risk of premature development of hypokinetic diseases'*?

   a) wellness

   b) physical fitness

   c) health-related physical fitness

   d) mental health

10.2 The World Health Organization defines what as *'a state of complete physical, mental and social well-being and not merely the absence of disease or infirmity'*?

   a) wellness

   b) physical fitness

   c) health-related fitness

   d) mental health

10.3 Cardiovascular endurance is also known as what?

   a) anaerobic capacity

   b) aerobic capacity

   c) ventilatory capacity

   d) respiratory capacity

10.4 $mlO_2.kg^{-1}min^{-1}$ is a measurement of what?

   a) anaerobic capacity

   b) lactate threshold

   c) VO_2 max

   d) OBLA

10.5 What are the benefits of regular cardiovascular training?

   a) increased HDL, increased exercise threshold, decreased heart rate for given intensity

   b) decreased HDL, increased exercise threshold, decreased heart rate for given intensity

   c) increased HDL, increased exercise threshold, increased heart rate for given intensity

   d) increased HDL, decreased exercise threshold, decreased heart rate for given intensity

10.6 What is the term used to define an increase in muscle cross-section?

   a) DOMS

   b) atrophy

    c) hypertrophy

    d) tone

10.7 What is the term used to define a decrease in muscle cross-section?

    a) DOMS

    b) atrophy

    c) hypertrophy

    d) tone

10.8 What are the benefits of regular resistance training?

    a) increased glucose tolerance, increased bone mass, increased resting metabolic rate

    b) increased glucose tolerance, increased bone mass, decreased resting metabolic rate

    c) decreased glucose tolerance, increased bone mass, increased resting metabolic rate

    d) increased glucose tolerance, decreased bone mass, increased resting metabolic rate

10.9 Strength gains in the first few weeks of a resistance training programme are usually due to what?

    a) hormonal changes

    b) muscular atrophy

    c) hypertrophy changes

    d) neural changes

10.10 What type of stretching involves the contraction of the agonist to elicit a stretch in the antagonist?

    a) static

    b) dynamic

    c) ballistic

    d) PNF

10.11 Which of the following formulae can be used to calculate BMI?

    a) $weight^2/height$

    b) $weight/height^2$

    c) $height/weight^2$

    d) $height^2/weight$

10.12 In relation to BMI, what figure is classed as obese?

    a) over 25

    b) over 30

    c) over 20

    d) over 15

Further reading

American College of Sports Medicine (2018) *ACSM Guidelines to Exercise Testing and Prescription* (10th ed.), Lippincott, Williams and Wilkins

Baechle, R.T. (2016) *Essentials of Strength Training and Conditioning* (4th ed.), Human Kinetics

Bird, S.P., Tarpenning, K.M. and Marino, F.E. (2005) 'Designing resistance training programmes to enhance muscular fitness: a review of the acute programme variables', *Sports Medicine*, 35: 841–851

Bompa, T.O. and Haff, G.G. (2009) *Periodisation Theory and Methodology of Training* (5th ed.), Human Kinetics

Bouchard, C., Blair, N.S., and Haskell, W. (2012) *Physical Activity, Fitness and Health* (2nd ed.), Human Kinetics

Boutcher, S.H. (2000) 'Cognitive performance, fitness and ageing', in Biddle, S.J.H., Fox, K.R. & Boutcher, S.H., *Physical Activity and Psychological Well-Being*, Routledge, 118–129

British Heart Foundation Health Promotion Research Group (2005) *Coronary Heart Disease Statistics*, University of Oxford: Department of Public Health

Department of Health (2000) *Coronary Heart Disease: National Service Framework for coronary heart disease – Modern standards and service models*, DoH

Department of Health (2004) *At Least 5 a Week: Evidence on the impact of physical activity and its relationship to health*, DoH

Department of Health, Health Survey for England (2007) *Healthy Lifestyles: Knowledge, attitudes and behaviour*, NHS Information Centre for Health and Social Care

Fleck, S.J. and Kraemer, W.J. (2014) *Designing Resistance Training Programs* (4th ed.), Human Kinetics

Howley, E.T. and Franks, B.D. (2003) *Health Fitness Instructor's Handbook* (4th ed.), Human Kinetics

Kugler, J., Seelbach, H. and Kruskemper, G.M. (1994) 'Effects of rehabilitation exercise programmes on anxiety and depression in coronary patients: a meta-analysis', *British Journal of Clinical Psychology*, 33: 401–410

Marieb, E.N. and Hoehn, K. (2011) *Human Anatomy and Physiology* (11th ed.), Pearson

McArdle, W.D., Katch, F.I. and Katch, V.L. (2007) *Exercise Physiology* (6th ed.), Lippincott, Williams & Wilkins

NHS information Centre, Lifestyle Statistics (2009) *Statistics on Obesity, Physical Activity and Diet: England, February 2009*, NHS Information Centre for Health and Social Care

Plisk, S.S. and Stone, M.H. (2003) 'Periodization strategies', *Strength and Conditioning Journal*, 25: 19–37

Ross, J.S. and Wilson, J.W. (2018) *Anatomy and Physiology in Health and Illness* (13th ed.), Churchill Livingstone

Schmidt, R.A. (2003) 'Motor schema theory after 27 years: reflections and implications for a new theory', *Research Quarterly for Exercise and Sport*, 74(4): 366–375

Sewell, D., Watkins, P. and Griffin, M. (2012) *Sport and Exercise Science: An Introduction* (2nd ed.), Hodder Arnold

Tortora, G.J. and Grabowski, S.R. (2017) *Principles of Anatomy and Physiology* (15th ed.), Wiley

Van Staa, T.P., Dennison, E.M., Leufkens, H.G. and Cooper, C. (2001) 'Epidemiology of fractures in England and Wales', *Bone*, 29: 517–522

Kenney, L., Wilmore, J.H. and Costhill, D.L. (2019) *Physiology of Sport and Exercise* (7th ed.), Human Kinetics

World Health Organization (2002) *The World Health Report 2002: Reducing risks, promoting healthy life*, WHO Press

PART 2

PRACTICAL APPLICATION

OF HEALTH

AND FITNESS

Part 2 looks at practical methods of applying the theory covered in Part 1. Each chapter provides example questions that are typical of industry-standard questions provided by accredited centres for the delivery of recognised qualifications. There is also a list of recommended reading for each chapter, should you wish to gain more in-depth knowledge of a particular subject area.

11 Screening for exercise and safety issues

OBJECTIVES

After completing this chapter, you will be able to:

1 Define the term 'screening' in relation to the health and fitness industry.

2 List and describe the different types of screening questionnaire available for the health and fitness industry.

3 Explain the term 'preparticipation health screening' and the process for using the screening algorithm proposed by the American College of Sports Medicine.

4 Briefly outline the areas of the Health and Safety at Work Act 1974 relating to the health and fitness industry.

5 Describe general issues relating to facility equipment management.

6 Describe procedures of risk assessment relating to hazards prior to exercise sessions.

7 Explain the procedure for dealing with an emergency situation during an exercise session.

8 Briefly outline the Health and Safety (First Aid) Regulations 1981 pertaining to the health and fitness industry.

9 Briefly discuss methods of reporting accidents and incidents.

10 Briefly discuss issues relating to child protection and how to seek further information.

Introduction

This chapter deals with various screening methods used within the health and fitness industry, as well as looking at safety issues in relation to guidelines within the Professional Standards framework for health and fitness. Instructors should be able to identify safety issues and describe methods of screening and the guidelines associated with these.

Later chapters in the book provide the knowledge required in relation to programme design, which, along with the content covered in this chapter, will provide you with the understanding and ability to design appropriate exercise programmes for apparently healthy individuals, in line with current guidelines for exercise.

Screening for exercise

One of the most important roles of a health and fitness instructor is to help individuals determine their current health and fitness status prior to undertaking a programme of exercise. Not only can this aid in planning and designing a safe and effective programme, but also in identifying any professional guidance that may be needed before the individual undertakes the programme. If any condition is identified which places the individual in a *particular population* category (see *Teaching Exercise to Special Populations* by Morc Coulson) and that the instructor is not qualified to deal with, they should inform the individual that this is the case and that they may only have a basic knowledge of the condition.

PREPARTICIPATION HEALTH SCREENING

The process of determining the health and fitness status of an individual is known as *preparticipation health screening*, normally shortened to *screening*. There are many ways in which screening can be carried out, such as that recommended by the American College of Sports Medicine (ACSM) 2018. The ACSM recommend the use of a preparticipation screening algorithm. The goals of this method of screening are to identify individuals:

a. Who should receive medical clearance before undertaking an exercise programme.
b. With clinically significant disease(s) who may benefit from a medically supervised exercise programme.
c. With medical conditions that may require exclusion from the programme.

The algorithm starts by classifying clients as those who DO or DO NOT participate in regular exercise (as described in Fig. 11.1).

The next stage is to identify those with known CV, metabolic or renal diseases or those with signs or symptoms suggestive of cardiac, peripheral vascular or cerebrovascular disease, Types 1 and 2 diabetes mellitus and renal

diseases as described in Fig. 11.1. Care should be taken by the instructor to screen for signs and symptoms that are described in Table 11.1.

Table 11.1 describes the major signs and symptoms related to the preparticipation algorithm. It is advised that instructors familiarise themselves with the terminology used. The final stage of the algorithm is to prescribe the appropriate exercise intensity for which guidelines are suggested on the bottom of the algorithm form. Medical clearance is sometimes warranted, however there is no universally accepted procedure therefore the instructor is encouraged to follow centre procedures or, if working as a sole trader, develop good communication links between themselves and local health care providers.

● **PAR-Q+** Instructors may prefer to use other methods of screening questionnaire, such as the *Physical Activity Readiness Questionnaire*, or *PAR-Q*, which was developed by the Canadian Society for Exercise Physiology. The current version, the PAR-Q+, is a questionnaire that can help to identify possible symptoms of cardiovascular, pulmonary and metabolic disease, as well as other conditions that might be aggravated by exercise. The form is self-explanatory and in certain circumstances where conditions are identified advises the individual to seek medical approval prior to undertaking a programme of exercise. If no conditions are identified, the form encourages a programme of light to moderate exercise to be undertaken at an intensity relevant to the current fitness level of the individual.

PAR-Q+ forms should be given out to all individuals and completed prior to the start of an exercise programme. The form should then be interpreted by a suitably qualified professional and dealt with in a confidential manner. If the instructor feels that the form reveals anything that is beyond the capacity of their training or experience, they should refer the case to a suitably qualified colleague or supervisor. It

TABLE 11.1

ACSM's major signs and symptoms suggestive of CV, metabolic and renal disease

Signs or symptoms	Clarification/significance
Pain; discomfort (or other angina equivalent) in the chest, neck, jaw or other areas that may result from myocardial ischaemia (blood flow to the heart is obstructed)	Key features favouring an ischaemic origin include the following: • *Character*: constricting, squeezing, burning, 'heaviness' feeling. • *Location*: substernal, across midthorax, anteriorly; in one or both arms, shoulders; in neck, cheeks, teeth; in forearms, fingers in interscapular region. • *Provoking factors*: exercise or exertion, excitement or other forms of stress, cold weather, occurrence after meals. Key features against an ischaemic origin include the following: • *Character*: dull ache, sharp stabbing jabs aggravated by breathing. • *Location*: in left submammary area; in left hemithorax. • *Provoking factors*: after completion of exercise, provoked by a specific body motion.
Shortness of breath at rest or with mild exertion	Dyspnoea (defined as abnormally uncomfortable awareness of breathing) is one of the principal systems of cardiac and pulmonary disease. It commonly occurs during strenuous exertion in healthy, well-trained individuals, and during moderate exertion in healthy, untrained individuals. It should be regarded as abnormal when it occurs at a level of exertion that is not expected to evoke this symptom in a given individual. Abnormal exertional dyspnoea suggests the presence of cardiopulmonary disorders; in particular, left ventricular dysfunction or chronic obstructive pulmonary disease.
Dizziness or syncope (fainting)	Syncope (defined as a loss of consciousness) is most commonly caused by a reduced perfusion of the brain. Dizziness and, in particular, syncope during exercise may result from cardiac disorders that prevent the normal rise (or an actual fall) in cardiac output. Such cardiac disorders are potentially life-threatening and include severe coronary artery disease, hypertrophic cardiomyopathy (the heart muscle thickens and makes it difficult to pump blood), aortic stenosis (narrowing of the aortic valve opening), and malignant ventricular arrhythmias (irregular contraction of the ventricles). Although dizziness or syncope shortly after cessation of exercise should not be ignored, these symptoms may occur even in healthy individuals as a result of a reduction in venous return (the return of de-oxygenated blood) to the heart.

TABLE 11.1 (CONTINUED)

ACSM's major signs and symptoms suggestive of CV, metabolic and renal disease

Orthopnoea (shortness of breath lying flat) or paroxysmal nocturnal dyspnoea (severe shortness of breath or coughing at night)	Orthopnoea refers to dyspnoea occurring at rest in the recumbent position that is relieved promptly by sitting upright or standing. Paroxysmal nocturnal dyspnoea refers to dyspnoea, beginning usually 2–5 hours after the onset of sleep, which may be relieved by sitting on the side of the bed or getting out of bed. Both are symptoms of left ventricular dysfunction. Although nocturnal dyspnoea may occur in individuals with chronic obstructive pulmonary disease (the term for a group of lung conditions not fully reversible), it differs in that it is usually relieved following a bowel movement rather than specifically by standing up.
Ankle oedema (swelling usually caused with fluid build-up)	Bilateral (both sides) ankle oedema that is most evident at night is a characteristic sign of heart failure or bilateral chronic venous insufficiency (problems with leg veins causing poor venous return). Unilateral oedema of a limb often results from venous thrombosis (blood clot) or lymphatic blockage (blockage of the lymph vessels that drain fluid from tissues in the body) in the limb. Generalised oedema (known as anasarca) occurs in individuals with the nephrotic syndrome (a collection of symptoms due to kidney damage), severe heart failure, or hepatic cirrhosis (liver damage).
Palpitations or tachycardia (resting heart rate over 100bpm)	Palpitations (defines as an unpleasant awareness of the forceful or rapid beating of the heart) may be induced by various disorders of cardiac rhythm. These include tachycardia (fast heart rate), bradycardia (slow heart rate) of sudden onset, ectopic beats (irregular rhythm), compensatory pauses (long pause after abnormal beat), and increased stroke volume resulting from valvular regurgitation (leaking valve). Palpitations often result from anxiety states and high cardiac output (or hyperkinetic) states, such as anaemia (iron deficiency in the blood), fever, thyrotoxicosis (effects of increased thyroid hormones), arteriovenous fistula (abnormal connection between an artery and vein), and the so-called idiopathic hyperkinetic heart syndrome (increased blood ejected each beat).

TABLE 11.1 (CONTINUED)

ACSM's major signs and symptoms suggestive of CV, metabolic and renal disease

Intermittent claudication (muscle pain normally in the legs on mild exertion)	Intermittent claudication refers to the pain that occurs in the lower extremities with an inadequate blood supply (usually as a result of atherosclerosis) that is brought on by exercise. The pain does not occur with standing or sitting, is reproducible from day to day, is more severe when walking upstairs or up a hill, and is often described as a cramp, which disappears within 1–2 minutes after stopping exercise. Coronary artery disease is more prevalent in individuals with intermittent claudication. Patients with diabetes are at increased risk for this condition.
Known heart murmur	Although some may be innocent, heart murmurs may indicate valvular or other cardiovascular disease. From an exercise safety standpoint, it is especially important to exclude hypertrophic cardiomyopathy and aortic stenosis as underlying causes because these are among the more common causes of exertion-related sudden cardiac death.
Unusual fatigue or shortness of breath with usual activities	Although there may be benign (not harmful in effect) origins for these symptoms, they also may signal the onset of or change in the status of cardiovascular disease or metabolic disease.

should also be noted that PAR-Q+ screening is normally only valid for a 12-month period.

• Physical activity screening questionnaires

Prior to designing a programme of exercise for an individual, it is recommended that previous and current client fitness levels are established. One of the methods commonly employed within the health and fitness industry is a *physical activity screening questionnaire*, which is often used to ensure the exercise programme is at the optimum level for the client. However, a fitness questionnaire is not a replacement for the PAR-Q+, but rather a supplement to it.

There is no accepted standard of fitness questionnaire available and many different types are used within the health and fitness industry. Typical questionnaires include the following questions:

1. Do you currently participate in any form of exercise?
2. How often do you participate in exercise?
3. What types of exercise do you currently participate in?
4. How long do you normally exercise for during each session?
5. Would you class your exercise as moderate or vigorous?

FIG. 11.1

ACSM preparticipation screening algorithm

Does **NOT** participate in regular exercise[1]			Participates in regular exercise[1]		
No CV[5], metabolic[6] or renal disease **AND** No signs or symptoms[7] suggestive of the above	Known CV[5], metabolic[6] or renal disease **AND** Asymptomatic	Any signs or symptoms[7] suggestive of CV[5], metabolic[6] or renal disease	No CV[5], metabolic[6] or renal disease **AND** No signs or symptoms[7] suggestive of the above	Known CV[5], metabolic[6] or renal disease **AND** Asymptomatic	Any signs or symptoms[7] suggestive of CV[5], metabolic[6] or renal disease
Medical clearance[8] not necessary	Medical clearance[8] recommended	Medical clearance[8] recommended	Medical clearance[8] not necessary	Medical clearance[8] for mod[3] intensity exercise not necessary. Medical clearance (within the last 12 months if no change in signs or symptoms) recommended before vigorous[4] exercise	Discontinue exercise and seek medical clearance[8]
Light[2] to mod[3] intensity exercise recommended. May gradually progress to vigorous[4]	Following medical clearance light[2] to mod[3] intensity exercise recommended. May gradually progress as tolerated following ACSM guidelines	Following medical clearance light[2] to mod[3] intensity exercise recommended. May gradually progress as tolerated following ACSM guidelines	Continue mod[3] or vigorous[4] intensity exercise. May gradually progress		May return to exercise following medical clearance[8]. Gradually progress as tolerated following ACSM guidelines
				Continue with mod[3] intensity exercise. Following medical clearance[8] may gradually progress as tolerated following ACSM guidelines.	

1 Exercise participation – Performing planned, structured activity at least 30 mins at moderate intensity on at least 3 days per week for at least the last 3 months.
2 Light intensity – 30–39% HRR (RPE 9–11) or an intensity that causes slight increases in HR and breathing.
3 Moderate intensity – 40–59% HRR (RPE 12–13) or an intensity that causes noticeable increases in HR and breathing.
4 Vigorous intensity – ≥60% HRR (RPE ≥14) or an intensity that causes substantial increases in HR and breathing.
5 CV disease – Cardiac, peripheral vascular, or cerebrovascular disease.
6 Metabolic disease – Type 1 and 2 diabetes mellitus.
7 Signs and symptoms – At rest or during activity. Includes pain, discomfort in the chest, neck, jaw, arms or any other areas that may result from ischemia; shortness of breath at rest or with mild exertion; dizziness; orthopnoea or paroxysmal nocturnal dyspnoea; ankle oedema; palpitations or tachycardia; intermittent claudication; known heart murmur; unusual fatigue or shortness of breath with usual activities.
8 Medical clearance – Approval from a health care professional to engage in exercise.

6. Can you walk briskly for 30 minutes without fatigue?
7. Can you jog for 20 minutes without fatigue?
8. What types of exercises do you enjoy doing?
9. What types of exercise do you not like doing?
10. If you do not currently exercise, when was the last time you participated in regular exercise?
11. How often did you participate in regular exercise and what type of exercise was it?

As with all information of a personal nature, the physical activity screening questionnaire must be treated confidentially. Confidentiality and other such values are explained in more detail within a set of standards known as the Code of Ethics. This applies to instructors within the health and fitness industry and constitutes a set of guidelines within which to work. For more details visit www.cimspa.co.uk

• **Lifestyle questionnaires** Lifestyle questionnaires are also commonly used in the health and fitness industry to elicit information about diet, exercise and activities regarded as *lifestyle activities*, such as walking, housework and

FIG. 11.2

Example of a PAR-Q+

Warburton D., Jamnik V., Bredin S., Shephard R., Gledhill N. (2019) The 2020 Physical Activity Readiness Questionnaire for Everyone (PAR-Q+) and electronic Physical Activity Readiness Medical Examination (ePARmed-X+). *Health & Fitness Journal of Canada* 12(4):58–61. https://doi.org/10.14288/hfjc.v12i4.295

2020 PAR-Q+

The Physical Activity Readiness Questionnaire for Everyone

The health benefits of regular physical activity are clear; more people should engage in physical activity every day of the week. Participating in physical activity is very safe for MOST people. This questionnaire will tell you whether it is necessary for you to seek further advice from your doctor OR a qualified exercise professional before becoming more physically active.

GENERAL HEALTH QUESTIONS

Please read the 7 questions below carefully and answer each one honestly: check YES or NO.	YES	NO
1) Has your doctor ever said that you have a heart condition ☐ **OR** high blood pressure ☐?	☐	☐
2) Do you feel pain in your chest at rest, during your daily activities of living, **OR** when you do physical activity?	☐	☐
3) Do you lose balance because of dizziness **OR** have you lost consciousness in the last 12 months? Please answer **NO** if your dizziness was associated with over-breathing (including during vigorous exercise).	☐	☐
4) Have you ever been diagnosed with another chronic medical condition (other than heart disease or high blood pressure)? **PLEASE LIST CONDITION(S) HERE:** _____	☐	☐
5) Are you currently taking prescribed medications for a chronic medical condition? **PLEASE LIST CONDITION(S) AND MEDICATIONS HERE:** _____	☐	☐
6) Do you currently have (or have had within the past 12 months) a bone, joint, or soft tissue (muscle, ligament, or tendon) problem that could be made worse by becoming more physically active? Please answer **NO** if you had a problem in the past, but it **does not limit your current ability** to be physically active. **PLEASE LIST CONDITION(S) HERE:** _____	☐	☐
7) Has your doctor ever said that you should only do medically supervised physical activity?	☐	☐

☑ **If you answered NO to all of the questions above, you are cleared for physical activity.**
Please sign the PARTICIPANT DECLARATION. You do not need to complete Pages 2 and 3.

- Start becoming much more physically active – start slowly and build up gradually.
- Follow Global Physical Activity Guidelines for your age (https://apps.who.int/iris/handle/10665/44399).
- You may take part in a health and fitness appraisal.
- If you are over the age of 45 yr and NOT accustomed to regular vigorous to maximal effort exercise, consult a qualified exercise professional before engaging in this intensity of exercise.
- If you have any further questions, contact a qualified exercise professional.

PARTICIPANT DECLARATION
If you are less than the legal age required for consent or require the assent of a care provider, your parent, guardian or care provider must also sign this form.

I, the undersigned, have read, understood to my full satisfaction and completed this questionnaire. I acknowledge that this physical activity clearance is valid for a maximum of 12 months from the date it is completed and becomes invalid if my condition changes. I also acknowledge that the community/fitness center may retain a copy of this form for its records. In these instances, it will maintain the confidentiality of the same, complying with applicable law.

NAME _____ DATE _____

SIGNATURE _____ WITNESS _____

SIGNATURE OF PARENT/GUARDIAN/CARE PROVIDER _____

⬤ **If you answered YES to one or more of the questions above, COMPLETE PAGES 2 AND 3.**

⚠ **Delay becoming more active if:**

- You have a temporary illness such as a cold or fever; it is best to wait until you feel better.
- You are pregnant - talk to your health care practitioner, your physician, a qualified exercise professional, and/or complete the ePARmed-X+ at www.eparmedx.com before becoming more physically active.
- Your health changes - answer the questions on Pages 2 and 3 of this document and/or talk to your doctor or a qualified exercise professional before continuing with any physical activity program.

FIG. 11.2 (CONTINUED)

Example of a PAR-Q+

2020 PAR-Q+

FOLLOW-UP QUESTIONS ABOUT YOUR MEDICAL CONDITION(S)

1. **Do you have Arthritis, Osteoporosis, or Back Problems?**
If the above condition(s) is/are present, answer questions 1a-1c   If **NO** ☐ go to question 2

1a.	Do you have difficulty controlling your condition with medications or other physician-prescribed therapies? (Answer **NO** if you are not currently taking medications or other treatments)	YES ☐ NO ☐
1b.	Do you have joint problems causing pain, a recent fracture or fracture caused by osteoporosis or cancer, displaced vertebra (e.g., spondylolisthesis), and/or spondylolysis/pars defect (a crack in the bony ring on the back of the spinal column)?	YES ☐ NO ☐
1c.	Have you had steroid injections or taken steroid tablets regularly for more than 3 months?	YES ☐ NO ☐

2. **Do you currently have Cancer of any kind?**
If the above condition(s) is/are present, answer questions 2a-2b   If **NO** ☐ go to question 3

2a.	Does your cancer diagnosis include any of the following types: lung/bronchogenic, multiple myeloma (cancer of plasma cells), head, and/or neck?	YES ☐ NO ☐
2b.	Are you currently receiving cancer therapy (such as chemotheraphy or radiotherapy)?	YES ☐ NO ☐

3. **Do you have a Heart or Cardiovascular Condition? This includes Coronary Artery Disease, Heart Failure, Diagnosed Abnormality of Heart Rhythm**
If the above condition(s) is/are present, answer questions 3a-3d   If **NO** ☐ go to question 4

3a.	Do you have difficulty controlling your condition with medications or other physician-prescribed therapies? (Answer **NO** if you are not currently taking medications or other treatments)	YES ☐ NO ☐
3b.	Do you have an irregular heart beat that requires medical management? (e.g., atrial fibrillation, premature ventricular contraction)	YES ☐ NO ☐
3c.	Do you have chronic heart failure?	YES ☐ NO ☐
3d.	Do you have diagnosed coronary artery (cardiovascular) disease and have not participated in regular physical activity in the last 2 months?	YES ☐ NO ☐

4. **Do you currently have High Blood Pressure?**
If the above condition(s) is/are present, answer questions 4a-4b   If **NO** ☐ go to question 5

4a.	Do you have difficulty controlling your condition with medications or other physician-prescribed therapies? (Answer **NO** if you are not currently taking medications or other treatments)	YES ☐ NO ☐
4b.	Do you have a resting blood pressure equal to or greater than 160/90 mmHg with or without medication? (Answer **YES** if you do not know your resting blood pressure)	YES ☐ NO ☐

5. **Do you have any Metabolic Conditions? This includes Type 1 Diabetes, Type 2 Diabetes, Pre-Diabetes**
If the above condition(s) is/are present, answer questions 5a-5e   If **NO** ☐ go to question 6

5a.	Do you often have difficulty controlling your blood sugar levels with foods, medications, or other physician-prescribed therapies?	YES ☐ NO ☐
5b.	Do you often suffer from signs and symptoms of low blood sugar (hypoglycemia) following exercise and/or during activities of daily living? Signs of hypoglycemia may include shakiness, nervousness, unusual irritability, abnormal sweating, dizziness or light-headedness, mental confusion, difficulty speaking, weakness, or sleepiness.	YES ☐ NO ☐
5c.	Do you have any signs or symptoms of diabetes complications such as heart or vascular disease and/or complications affecting your eyes, kidneys, **OR** the sensation in your toes and feet?	YES ☐ NO ☐
5d.	Do you have other metabolic conditions (such as current pregnancy-related diabetes, chronic kidney disease, or liver problems)?	YES ☐ NO ☐
5e.	Are you planning to engage in what for you is unusually high (or vigorous) intensity exercise in the near future?	YES ☐ NO ☐

FIG. 11.2 (CONTINUED)

Example of a PAR-Q+

2020 PAR-Q+

6. **Do you have any Mental Health Problems or Learning Difficulties?** This includes Alzheimer's, Dementia, Depression, Anxiety Disorder, Eating Disorder, Psychotic Disorder, Intellectual Disability, Down Syndrome

If the above condition(s) is/are present, answer questions 6a-6b   If **NO** ☐ go to question 7

		YES	NO
6a.	Do you have difficulty controlling your condition with medications or other physician-prescribed therapies? (Answer **NO** if you are not currently taking medications or other treatments)	☐	☐
6b.	Do you have Down Syndrome **AND** back problems affecting nerves or muscles?	☐	☐

7. **Do you have a Respiratory Disease?** This includes Chronic Obstructive Pulmonary Disease, Asthma, Pulmonary High Blood Pressure

If the above condition(s) is/are present, answer questions 7a-7d   If **NO** ☐ go to question 8

		YES	NO
7a.	Do you have difficulty controlling your condition with medications or other physician-prescribed therapies? (Answer **NO** if you are not currently taking medications or other treatments)	☐	☐
7b.	Has your doctor ever said your blood oxygen level is low at rest or during exercise and/or that you require supplemental oxygen therapy?	☐	☐
7c.	If asthmatic, do you currently have symptoms of chest tightness, wheezing, laboured breathing, consistent cough (more than 2 days/week), or have you used your rescue medication more than twice in the last week?	☐	☐
7d.	Has your doctor ever said you have high blood pressure in the blood vessels of your lungs?	☐	☐

8. **Do you have a Spinal Cord Injury?** This includes Tetraplegia and Paraplegia

If the above condition(s) is/are present, answer questions 8a-8c   If **NO** ☐ go to question 9

		YES	NO
8a.	Do you have difficulty controlling your condition with medications or other physician-prescribed therapies? (Answer **NO** if you are not currently taking medications or other treatments)	☐	☐
8b.	Do you commonly exhibit low resting blood pressure significant enough to cause dizziness, light-headedness, and/or fainting?	☐	☐
8c.	Has your physician indicated that you exhibit sudden bouts of high blood pressure (known as Autonomic Dysreflexia)?	☐	☐

9. **Have you had a Stroke?** This includes Transient Ischemic Attack (TIA) or Cerebrovascular Event

If the above condition(s) is/are present, answer questions 9a-9c   If **NO** ☐ go to question 10

		YES	NO
9a.	Do you have difficulty controlling your condition with medications or other physician-prescribed therapies? (Answer **NO** if you are not currently taking medications or other treatments)	☐	☐
9b.	Do you have any impairment in walking or mobility?	☐	☐
9c.	Have you experienced a stroke or impairment in nerves or muscles in the past 6 months?	☐	☐

10. **Do you have any other medical condition not listed above or do you have two or more medical conditions?**

If you have other medical conditions, answer questions 10a-10c   If **NO** ☐ read the Page 4 recommendations

		YES	NO
10a.	Have you experienced a blackout, fainted, or lost consciousness as a result of a head injury within the last 12 months **OR** have you had a diagnosed concussion within the last 12 months?	☐	☐
10b.	Do you have a medical condition that is not listed (such as epilepsy, neurological conditions, kidney problems)?	☐	☐
10c.	Do you currently live with two or more medical conditions?	☐	☐

PLEASE LIST YOUR MEDICAL CONDITION(S) AND ANY RELATED MEDICATIONS HERE: _____

_____

GO to Page 4 for recommendations about your current medical condition(s) and sign the PARTICIPANT DECLARATION.

FIG. 11.2 (CONTINUED)

Example of a PAR-Q+

2020 PAR-Q+

☑ **If you answered NO to all of the FOLLOW-UP questions (pgs. 2-3) about your medical condition, you are ready to become more physically active - sign the PARTICIPANT DECLARATION below:**

- It is advised that you consult a qualified exercise professional to help you develop a safe and effective physical activity plan to meet your health needs.

- You are encouraged to start slowly and build up gradually - 20 to 60 minutes of low to moderate intensity exercise, 3-5 days per week including aerobic and muscle strengthening exercises.

- As you progress, you should aim to accumulate 150 minutes or more of moderate intensity physical activity per week.

- If you are over the age of 45 yr and **NOT** accustomed to regular vigorous to maximal effort exercise, consult a qualified exercise professional before engaging in this intensity of exercise.

● **If you answered YES to one or more of the follow-up questions about your medical condition:**

You should seek further information before becoming more physically active or engaging in a fitness appraisal. You should complete the specially designed online screening and exercise recommendations program - the **ePARmed-X+ at www.eparmedx.com** and/or visit a qualified exercise professional to work through the ePARmed-X+ and for further information.

⚠ **Delay becoming more active if:**

✓ You have a temporary illness such as a cold or fever; it is best to wait until you feel better.

✓ You are pregnant - talk to your health care practitioner, your physician, a qualified exercise professional, and/or complete the ePARmed-X+ **at www.eparmedx.com** before becoming more physically active.

✓ Your health changes - talk to your doctor or qualified exercise professional before continuing with any physical activity program.

- You are encouraged to photocopy the PAR-Q+. You must use the entire questionnaire and NO changes are permitted.
- The authors, the PAR-Q+ Collaboration, partner organizations, and their agents assume no liability for persons who undertake physical activity and/or make use of the PAR-Q+ or ePARmed-X+. If in doubt after completing the questionnaire, consult your doctor prior to physical activity.

PARTICIPANT DECLARATION

- All persons who have completed the PAR-Q+ please read and sign the declaration below.

- If you are less than the legal age required for consent or require the assent of a care provider, your parent, guardian or care provider must also sign this form.

I, the undersigned, have read, understood to my full satisfaction and completed this questionnaire. I acknowledge that this physical activity clearance is valid for a maximum of 12 months from the date it is completed and becomes invalid if my condition changes. I also acknowledge that the community/fitness center may retain a copy of this form for records. In these instances, it will maintain the confidentiality of the same, complying with applicable law.

NAME _____   DATE _____

SIGNATURE _____   WITNESS _____

SIGNATURE OF PARENT/GUARDIAN/CARE PROVIDER _____

──── For more information, please contact ────
www.eparmedx.com
Email: eparmedx@gmail.com

Citation for PAR-Q+
Warburton DER, Jamnik VK, Bredin SSD, and Gledhill N on behalf of the PAR-Q+ Collaboration. The Physical Activity Readiness Questionnaire for Everyone (PAR-Q+) and Electronic Physical Activity Readiness Medical Examination (ePARmed-X+). Health & Fitness Journal of Canada 4(2):3-23, 2011.

Key References
1. Jamnik VK, Warburton DER, Makarski J, McKenzie DC, Shephard RJ, Stone J, and Gledhill N. Enhancing the effectiveness of clearance for physical activity participation; background and overall process. APNM 36(S1):S3-S13, 2011.
2. Warburton DER, Gledhill N, Jamnik VK, Bredin SSD, McKenzie DC, Stone J, Charlesworth S, and Shephard RJ. Evidence-based risk assessment and recommendations for physical activity clearance; Consensus Document. APNM 36(S1):S266-s298, 2011.
3. Chisholm DM, Collis ML, Kulak LL, Davenport W, and Gruber N. Physical activity readiness. British Columbia Medical Journal. 1975;17:375-378.
4. Thomas S, Reading J, and Shephard RJ. Revision of the Physical Activity Readiness Questionnaire (PAR-Q). Canadian Journal of Sport Science 1992;17:4 338-345.

The PAR-Q+ was created using the evidence-based AGREE process (1) by the PAR-Q+ Collaboration chaired by Dr. Darren E. R. Warburton with Dr. Norman Gledhill, Dr. Veronica Jamnik, and Dr. Donald C. McKenzie (2). Production of this document has been made possible through financial contributions from the Public Health Agency of Canada and the BC Ministry of Health Services. The views expressed herein do not necessarily represent the views of the Public Health Agency of Canada or the BC Ministry of Health Services.

gardening. Lifestyle activities have been shown to have numerous health benefits and can be integrated into a typical daily lifestyle for most individuals, and these types of questionnaires can help instructors to identify areas of lifestyle that could be improved and could be incorporated into an overall programme of exercise. It must be stressed, however, that recommendations relating to diet are limited by national occupational standards and advice beyond this should only be given by those who are qualified in this area.

As with physical activity screening questionnaires, lifestyle questionnaires are not a replacement for the PAR-Q+ but a supplement to it. Many lifestyle questionnaires are in use in the health and fitness industry, but typical questionnaires include the following questions:

1. Do you currently smoke and, if so, how much?
2. Do you drink alcohol and, if so, how much on average each week?
3. Do you work at a desk each day?
4. How do you travel to work?
5. What do you do at break times?
6. Are there any stairs at your place of work?
7. What is your typical daily routine?
8. How far do you walk on a typical day?
9. Would you consider yourself to have a healthy diet?
10. Do you snack between meals?
11. When do you have your last meal of the day?

Note: With all pre-exercise questionnaires, the instructor must respect the confidentiality of all written material relating to client information by ensuring safe storage and private access.

VERBAL SCREENING

In addition to the PAR-Q+ screening form, instructors can screen clients verbally prior to an exercise session. A certain amount of time

may have elapsed between a client completing a PAR-Q+ and actually beginning a programme of exercise. Within this period of time injuries may have occurred, so individuals should be asked if they know of any reason why they should not exercise or if they have any current injury that could prevent them from exercising. In certain facilities, it is also possible for members to access studio classes without going through the screening process. For this reason, when supervising a one-to-one or group exercise session, it is advisable to carry out verbal screening prior to the start of the session.

It is at the instructor's discretion to decide whether any response warrants medical referral. All GP surgeries have their own procedure for exercise referral, so it is important to be aware of the procedures employed at geographically relevant surgeries. Verbal screening is also confidential, therefore discretion must be used in a group exercise situation.

Note: Some health and fitness facilities use an informed consent form that individuals agree to and sign before undertaking an exercise programme. These forms state the benefits and risks associated with exercise and are intended as a precaution against liability.

TASK
List the types of screening available to instructors and describe the benefits of each.

Health and safety issues

It is important for health and fitness instructors to be aware that they need to address the many potential health and safety issues due to the emerging litigational environment that they work in and, more importantly, for the safety of their clients. The main areas that instructors should be aware of are health and safety at work, equipment management, risk assessment, emergency first aid, potential accidents/incidents and child protection.

HEALTH AND SAFETY AT WORK

As in any environment, health and safety is an issue in any facility in which exercise is undertaken. The Health and Safety at Work Act (HSWA) 1974 outlines the role of the instructor (as well as those appointed persons for all areas of health and safety) in relation to prevention of accidents and, although the HSWA is an extensive document, a selection of the roles relevant to the health and fitness instructor are as follows:

1. Take responsible care for their own safety and that of others.
2. Co-operate with employers in matters of safety.
3. Do not interfere with or misuse anything provided for safety.

Larger health and fitness organisations should, by law, make a health and safety policy statement available to all staff and provide employees with relevant training. However, prior to working in any health and fitness environment the instructor must be familiar with several fundamental safety issues. It is in the interest of the instructor to identify and familiarise himself with the normal operating procedures (NOPs) (this often includes such things as security procedures and day-to-day operations) and emergency operating procedures (EOPs) (such as fire and medical emergency) in the workplace to become aware of procedures that could help to minimise the occurrence of accident or injury. If an instructor is unsure of any health and safety concern, they should always contact their

immediate line supervisor in order to clarify the issue. This is also the case should an instructor feel that procedures do not reflect health and safety regulations in some way.

EQUIPMENT MANAGEMENT

The management of equipment during an exercise session is important with respect to overall safety. Equipment should not form an obstruction to the participants who are in the facility. For example, free weights should always be returned to their correct storage rack. It is also important to check equipment, such as pulleys and cables, for any wear and tear or malfunction prior to use. Instructors should also know how to operate any equipment and be able to locate manufacturers' manuals or guides. These guides should indicate the type and frequency of maintenance required. The facilities guidelines for the use of equipment are usually found in the NOPs, along with relevant paperwork such as gym maintenance report sheets and faulty equipment notices.

RISK ASSESSMENT

The statutory framework relating to risk management and health and safety at work in the UK is mainly covered by the Management of Health and Safety at Work Regulations (1999); this document states that all self-employed persons should carry out risk assessment to identify health and safety risks to clients. All health and fitness facilities have hazards and risks therefore it is the purpose of risk assessment to identify any that might be present. Hazards can come in the form of equipment left lying around or substances that are used for cleaning, etc., that are not stored or used correctly. In this case there is guidance in the form of Control of Substances Hazardous to Health Regulations, which all facilities should have. Certain exercises can also constitute a risk

FIG. 11.3

Example risk assessment form

Potential risk	Method of minimising risk	Action to be taken	Done
Recovery from shoulder injury	Limit range of motion and weight	Set pec dec range to start at limited range of motion	✓
Trips due to free weights on floor in gym area	Ensure members return free weights to storage when finished	Put up signs around gym area to instruct members to return free weights	✓
Slippage on floor space around water fountain	Wipe floor regularly with paper towel	Add this to daily cleaning rota	✓

depending on the individual concerned in terms of injury or disability. Although risks cannot be eradicated completely, they can be recognised, addressed and minimised. When planning an exercise session, it is advisable to complete and document a risk assessment. This acts as a written reminder for the instructor as well as providing evidence that preventative steps were taken, should an accident occur. Fig. 11.3 provides a template that can be used to formulate and document a basic risk assessment.

EMERGENCY SITUATIONS

As mentioned previously, instructors should be familiar with the facility's EOPs and how to report them. If problems occur during any emergency (such as a fire exit was locked), this should also be reported by the instructor to the appointed facility health and safety officer. If an emergency occurs during an exercise session, the instructor should follow the procedure below:

1. Assess the situation. Approach quickly but remain calm as casualties are often in distress. Identify any risks to yourself, the casualties and bystanders.
2. Make the area safe. The conditions that caused the emergency may need to be made safe.
3. Give emergency aid. Assess the casualty and give first aid.
4. Get help. Send someone for help or telephone for assistance.
5. Comfort and reassure the casualty until help arrives.

When contacting the emergency services, clear and accurate information must be given with regard to the following:

- Own name
- Nature of emergency
- Details of any casualty
- Time of emergency

- Facility details
- Contact number

FIRST AID

Prior to the arrival of the emergency services, the instructor must deal with the emergency in the correct manner. Any requirement for emergency first aid must be given and any minor injuries (such as cuts, sprains, strains) can be dealt with accordingly; the casualty must be made as comfortable as possible. All staff at the centre must be informed about the arrival of the emergency services so that clear access can be prepared in advance. As a simple guideline, the following procedure should be adhered to during an emergency situation:

1. Inform the people involved about the correct emergency procedures.
2. Follow procedures in a calm but correct manner.
3. Maintain the safety of those involved at all times.
4. Clearly and accurately report any problems to a responsible colleague.
5. Make a detailed report of the incident afterwards.

According to the Health and Safety (First Aid) Regulations 1981, employers must provide adequate equipment and facilities to enable first aid to be carried out on sick or injured employees. This does not by law extend to customers using the facility, although instructors trained in first aid should make every attempt to administer first aid, should the situation arise. A current first-aid certificate is required before acceptance onto the Register of Exercise Professionals. Also, facilities should have a visible notice of the details of any first aider on site.

ACCIDENT/INCIDENT REPORT

In the event of an accident or incident during a gym session in which the instructor is in charge, an accident/incident report must be completed as a record of the event. The facility at which the instructor is working must provide the relevant form. It is important that this form is completed at the earliest available opportunity so that an accurate recall of the event can be made.

Child and vulnerable adult protection

According to Her Majesty's Government, any adult who works with children has a responsibility to keep them safe and protect them from sexual, physical and emotional harm. Failure to do this could be regarded as neglect and could lead to prosecution. For full details regarding duty of care go to www.everychildmatters.gov.uk. Key aspects of legislation have recently been extended to include similar standards of protection to 'vulnerable adults'. A vulnerable adult is defined by the UK government as 'a person aged 18 years or over who is in receipt or need of community care services by reason of mental or other disability, age, or illness and who is unable to take care of themselves or protect themselves against significant harm or exploitation'. In 1999 the Protection of Children Act was implemented with a view to increase the level of protection for children by screening those wishing to supervise children (not just in an exercise scenario) in order to identify those deemed not suitable to do so. For example, those deemed unsuitable would be people whose names appeared on the following lists:

TABLE 11.2

Summary of areas of duty of care

AREA	MAIN POINTS	ADVICE	INFORMATION
Confidentiality	Treat all information as confidential Do not allow others access to this information	Keep confidential information in a lockable place	Data Protection Act 1998
Sexual conduct	ALL sexual activity is a criminal offence Special attention can be construed as grooming Report any concerns about infatuation	Never make sexual remarks or jokes Never discuss your own relationship. Always make contact by email or phone through the parent or guardian Avoid having favourites and giving special attention	Sexual Offences Act 2003 Working Together to Safeguard Children: 2006 HM Government
Social contact	Social contact between trainers and vulnerable clients is not encouraged Trainers should never invite vulnerable clients to their homes	Make supervisors aware of any social contact with vulnerable clients and their families Never allow vulnerable clients into your home without their parents	
Communication	This includes phones, emails, websites and cameras Contact only in professional instances, such as informing that a session is cancelled	Always communicate through the parent or guardian Always get written permission for photos or videos	Code of Conduct

TABLE 11.2 (CONTINUED)

Summary of areas of duty of care

AREA	MAIN POINTS	ADVICE	INFORMATION
Physical contact	Physical contact is often required in instructing as long as it is appropriate Some vulnerable clients may feel uncomfortable about this whereas others may initiate inappropriate contact There may be cultural or religious issues	Get permission from vulnerable clients before any contact Try to keep parents informed of the need for this contact in instructing Make sure vulnerable clients know of the boundaries Report any issues immediately	Code of Conduct
Comforting	Vulnerable clients often become distressed for many reasons, especially younger children Some vulnerable clients may use this to seek comfort Professional judgement is key	Often a hand on the shoulder is enough to comfort Never comfort in a one-to-one situation unless another trainer or parent is present Record any issues you may be unsure about	

- List 99 from The Department of Education And Skills (DfES)
- Protection of Children Act list
- Protection of Vulnerable Adults list
- Department of Health list

The intention of the Act is that anyone wishing to deliver children's activities is required to carry out a disclosure check, which cross-references lists such as those above. To cater for this, the Home Office set up an organisation called the Criminal Records Bureau to deal with the checks. In the fitness industry the term 'safeguarding' is commonly used. Safeguarding can be thought of as the wide approach to meeting the needs of all children and vulnerable adults (including those who may be at risk from abuse). All those directly or indirectly involved with children's and vulnerable adults' leisure activities have a responsibility to:

- Review their own practice in situations to ensure that they are complying with recognised codes of conduct.
- Recognise the signs and symptoms and indicators of abuse and the impact this has on children and vulnerable adults.

- Respond in an appropriate way and take appropriate action if concerns are raised.

Safeguarding and protection of children and vulnerable adults covers many areas, such as physical contact, confidentiality, sexual conduct, social contact, communication and comforting, as outlined in Table 11.2.

When training within a gym environment with children or vulnerable adults the instructor should be aware that they are in 'loco parentis'. This means that in this situation it is their responsibility to ensure the individuals are using the correct and suitable equipment according to their ability and mental capacity.

In this environment it is crucial that the instructor understands their responsibilities and limitations. It is important therefore to demonstrate safeguarding behaviour at all times; this includes:

- Acting as a role model.
- Adhering to the policies and procedures.
- Adhering to the code of practice.
- Always wearing uniform and/or a name badge if one is provided.
- Understanding and acting upon their responsibilities.
- Recognising the need to protect the rights of participation, for fun, enjoyment and achievement for all.
- Reporting any suspected abuse to the safeguarding and protection officer or senior manager.
- Responding to cases of abuse in a responsible manner.
- Working in an open environment.

Children can often become infatuated with instructor figures, which can sometimes be misconstrued as affection and lead to potential grooming and sexual abuse. Instructors should be aware of this and try to give equal attention to all children in a group situation and follow the golden rule of never being alone with children. Situations sometimes arise when a child approaches an instructor and divulges sensitive information about potential abuse by another adult. Even though this puts the instructor in a very delicate situation, it is not their responsibility to decide if child abuse or inappropriate behaviour has taken place. Therefore the incident must be reported immediately but confidentially, as not all accusations turn out to be true. All facilities should have relevant reporting procedures as not all instructors will feel confident in this area, so they should be aware of who they should discuss concerns with and the limit of their own involvement. Organisations usually have a welfare protection officer or a line manager but if the child or vulnerable adult chooses the instructor as their 'trusted' contact then the following guidelines should be followed:

- Stay calm, reassure, listen and let the person talk.
- Do not promise to keep secrets.
- Do not interrogate or ask leading questions.
- Do not approach the alleged abuser, or the parents/carer of the person.
- Record in writing the details of what has been said, heard or seen.

There are also simple steps an instructor can take to protect themselves from accusations of abuse such as:

- Work in an open environment, avoiding spending time alone with children and/or vulnerable adults.
- Never take photographs of children and young people without the permission of the parents, carers and the facility operators.
- Always consider your behaviour towards children and vulnerable adults.
- Always take action if you have a concern about the behaviour of an adult or child towards another child or vulnerable adult.

- Promote the welfare of your clients, even if this means letting another professional take over.
- Never engage in intimacy with vulnerable people including immediately after instructing a session has ended.

If the instructor requires advice for any reason then they should contact:

- NSPCC Child Protection Helpline on 0808 800 5000, or
- ChildLine on 0800 1111

Abuse can take many forms, such as physical, emotional, neglect, bullying and sexual, and is often difficult to identify. Table 11.3 gives a brief outline of the areas of abuse and typical physical and behavioural signs.

TABLE 11.3

Physical and behavioural signs of abuse

Abuse area	Physical signs	Behavioural signs
Physical	• Unexplained bruising/hand marks, burns, breaks, scalds	• Flinching, covering up, reluctance to see GP • Depressed, withdrawn, aggressive outbursts
Emotional	• Speech disorders • Lack of progress • Sudden weight gain or loss	• Self-harm, fear of making mistakes • Doesn't take part, strange behaviour • Drop in self-esteem
Neglect	• Always hungry, underweight • Poorly dressed, unclean	• Always tired and late • Loner, no chaperone
Bullying	• Stomach and headaches • Scratching and bruising	• Mood swings, can't concentrate • Poor performance, won't engage, withdrawn
Sexual	• Walking discomfort • Genital itching • Signs of self-harm	• Self-harm, no friends, sexual actions • Change in behaviour, fear of people • Eating disorders, having secrets

EXAMPLE QUESTIONS

11.1 The PAR-Q+ is a screening questionnaire used to identify conditions prior to encouraging exercise at:

a) a vigorous level

b) a high intensity

c) a light-to-moderate intensity

d) all levels

11.2 The PAR-Q+ is a screening questionnaire that is valid for what period of time?

a) no time limit

b) six weeks

c) six months

d) 12 months

11.3 True or false? The PAR-Q+ is a confidential document.

True   False

11.4 Which of the following best describes the term 'myocardial ischaemia'?

a) another term for heart attack

b) obstruction of blood flow to the heart

c) defective heart valve

d) bleeding from the heart muscle

11.5 Which of the following best describes the term 'dyspnoea'?

a) pain in the lower extremities

b) fluid build-up

c) abnormal heart rhythm

d) abnormally uncomfortable awareness of breathing

11.6 Which of the following best describes the term 'tachycardia'?

a) heart rate response to exercise

b) abnormal heart rhythm

c) resting heart rate below 60bpm

d) resting heart rate over 100bpm

11.7 Which of the following best describes the term 'bradycardia'?

a) heart rate response to exercise

b) abnormal heart rhythm

c) resting heart rate below 60bpm

d) resting heart rate over 100bpm

11.8 Which of the following best describes the term 'oedema'?

a) swelling usually caused with fluid build-up

b) abnormal heart rhythm

c) pain in the lower extremities

d) abnormally uncomfortable awareness of breathing

11.9 Which of the following best describes the term 'claudication'?

a) swelling usually caused with fluid build-up

b) abnormal heart rhythm

c) pain in the lower extremities

d) abnormally uncomfortable awareness of breathing

11.10 Which of the following best describes the term 'orthopnoea'?

a) high levels of carbon dioxide in the blood

b) abnormally uncomfortable awareness of breathing

c) shortness of breath lying flat

d) airways obstruction

11.11 The Health and Safety at Work Act (HSWA) 1974 outlines which of the following as roles of the instructor?

a) take responsible care for their own safety and that of others

b) co-operate with employers in matters of safety

c) both A and B

d) neither A nor B

11.12 True or false? The Health and Safety (First Aid) Regulations 1981 states that employers are required to provide adequate equipment and facilities to enable first aid to be carried out on employees but not necessarily customers using the facility.

True   False

Further reading

American College of Sports Medicine (2018) *ACSM Guidelines to Exercise Testing and Prescription* (10th ed.), Lippincott, Williams & Wilkins

Baechle, R.T. (2016) *Essentials of Strength Training and Conditioning* (4th ed.), Human Kinetics

HM Government (2003) *Every Child Matters*, HMSO

HM Government (2004) *Children Act 2004*, HMSO

HM Government (2006) *Working Together to Safeguard Children: A guide to inter-agency working to safeguard and promote the welfare of children*, HMSO

Howley, E.T. and Franks, B.D. (2003) *Health Fitness Instructor's Handbook* (4th ed.) Human Kinetics

Sewell, D., Watkins, P. and Griffin, M. (2012) *Sport and Exercise Science: An Introduction* (2nd ed.), Hodder Arnold

12 Behavioural Change and Goal Setting

OBJECTIVES

After completing this chapter, you will be able to:

1 Describe the role and responsibilities of the instructor.
2 Briefly discuss psychology in relation to exercise.
3 List and describe the stages of the Prochaska and DiClemente Stages of Change Model.
4 List and describe the cognitive and behavioural processes relating to the Stages of Change Model.
5 Relate the cognitive and behavioural processes to the appropriate stage of change.
6 List various motivational factors relating to individuals initiating or maintaining an exercise programme.
7 Explain how goal setting can be used in an exercise environment.
8 Describe the Balance of Good Health Plate Model in relation to healthy eating and relating to government key messages.
9 Describe the functions of certain nutrients including fluid, minerals and vitamins.
10 Briefly describe what is meant by the energy equation.

Introduction

This chapter deals with the roles and responsibilities of the instructor within the guidelines of the Code of Ethical Practice. It also deals with common processes of behavioural change and goal-setting strategies in relation to guidelines within the Professional Standards framework for health and fitness. Within this framework, instructors should be able to identify and describe common processes of behavioural change, as well as describe general methods of goal setting within the health and fitness industry.

Later chapters in the book provide information about programme design that, along with the content covered in this chapter, provides the instructor with the understanding and ability to design appropriate exercise programmes for apparently healthy individuals, in line with current guidelines for exercise.

Role and responsibilities of the instructor

One of the main roles of the fitness professional is to help make small but lasting changes to people's lifestyles. Poor diet and inactivity have been linked to the risk of developing disease, such as coronary heart disease, hypertension, stroke, obesity, diabetes, cancers and many other conditions, yet despite the well-documented health benefits of a physically active lifestyle, much of the adult population remains sedentary. For this reason, the government has highlighted in many of its 'Health of a Nation' documents the need for a change in people's diet and exercise habits. In order to address this overarching role, instructors should be mindful of the responsibilities they have as fitness professionals.

DEVELOP THE INSTRUCTOR–CLIENT RELATIONSHIP

The instructor must develop a relationship of trust with clients. A client is more likely to adhere to an exercise programme if they have trust in what the instructor is telling them.

DEFINE WORKING BOUNDARIES

When working with a new client, it is important that they are made fully aware of exactly what they can and can't do. As part of the fitness Code of Ethics, an instructor should always inform a client that should a service be needed that is outside the range of the instructor's skills, they may refer them to another health professional.

VALUE THE CLIENT

One of the clear messages within the Code of Ethical Practice relates to valuing all clients equally (referred to as valuing diversity) regardless of their class, gender, sexuality, culture, religion or race. It is important that instructors value all clients equally and adapt their service to the specific needs of each client as far as it is practically possible in order to avoid potential discrimination that clients might experience. For example, there are certain religions such as Islam where it is considered inappropriate for females to exercise, therefore, if a male instructor is faced with this situation, exercise sessions behind closed doors with a female instructor should be offered.

MAINTAIN CONFIDENTIALITY

In the context of gym instruction, confidentiality relates to keeping any information that is passed between two persons (instructor–client or instructor–colleague) confidential and not shared with others without permission. As long as instructors adhere to the Code of Ethical Practice, confidentiality will not be a cause for concern.

FAMILIARISATION WITH THE CODE OF ETHICAL PRACTICE

Instructors should familiarise themselves with the areas of the Code of Ethical Practice. In the health and fitness industry, this code outlines good practice in four main areas: rights, relationships, responsibilities and standards. When joining the Register of Exercise Professionals, instructors assent to abide by this code and in turn accept their responsibility to themselves; to people who participate in exercise; to other fitness professionals and colleagues; to their respective fitness associations, professional bodies and institutes; to their employer; and to society. In the unfortunate event of a client complaint, the instructor should always remain professional in the way with which they deal with it.

A scheduled meeting with the client and another unbiased professional colleague can often be enough to resolve minor complaints (but, however small, make sure they are recorded in note form or audio format and a copy given to all parties). In more serious cases of alleged professional misconduct or failure to comply with the terms of membership of the register, clients making the complaint can be referred to the Professional Practice Committee of the Fitness Alliance, which will consider any need for sanctions. Guidance from the committee could also be sought in cases where disagreement or conflict between colleagues cannot be resolved. However, every effort should be made to resolve a disagreement between colleagues before contacting the committee.

PRESENT A POSITIVE IMAGE

As a fitness professional, it is important to present a positive image of one's self. Opinions are often formed within the first few seconds of meeting someone for the first time, which means first impressions are vital. The instructor therefore should act in a professional manner at all times. The acronym PEAP should help the instructor to do this:

P – Polite: say hello and introduce yourself and state your name
E – Eye contact: maintain eye contact at all times
A – Appearance: be professional in your appearance and set an example
P – Person's name: listen carefully and remember the name of the person

Exercise psychology

As well as the physiological benefits of exercise, there are many psychological benefits that play an important part in helping individuals to take up and maintain a regular programme of exercise. The psychological effects of exercise can be difficult to measure; however, it is claimed anecdotally that exercise can improve subjective feelings such as self-esteem, mood, self-image and confidence. It is also thought that exercise can help to reduce stress and anxiety by providing a distraction.

Even though there are possible physiological explanations for these psychological effects, such as endorphins released after exercise having a positive effect on mood, psychological strategies about exercise are considered to play an important role in uptake and adherence to exercise. One of the main areas of focus from a psychological perspective is finding strategies to help individuals overcome barriers to exercise by making permanent changes to their lifestyle and behaviour. These barriers include lack of funds, poor self-image, lack of enjoyment and, primarily, lack of available time. Instructors within the health and fitness industry might choose to identify which barriers to exercise are relevant to their particular client by simply asking direct questions. Once these barriers have been identified, the instructor can devise strategies to help overcome them. For example, if lack of time is an issue, the instructor could suggest walking more briskly whenever there is a need to walk, or getting off the bus one stop earlier if the client uses public transport. The instructor could also choose to use psychological strategies that have been successful following many years of research. One such strategy is the Behavioural Change Model discussed below.

Behavioural change

Much of the adult population does not engage in any form of regular exercise; therefore, starting an exercise programme often requires a change in lifestyle and habits on the part of the individual. This is otherwise known as *behavioural change*. It can be challenging for both the individual and the instructor to overcome habits that have been in place for many years, as research has suggested that behavioural change is a long-term process. However, models such as Prochaska and DiClemente's *Stages of Change Model* can help instructors to facilitate the process.

STAGES OF CHANGE MODEL

This model proposes that there are a number of stages to any lifestyle change, such as stopping smoking or alcohol rehabilitation. Indeed, the research carried out by Prochaska and DiClemente used smoking cessation as the theme for the conception of the model; however, it can also be applied to exercise uptake.

As can be seen from Fig. 12.1, there are several stages of change that will vary in duration depending on the individual. Table 12.1 describes the stages of change in more detail.

It is interesting to note that stages of change in relation to exercise uptake are cyclical in nature: in other words, an individual can go from one stage to the next and back again without ever moving any further on in the model. Approximately 15 per cent of all individuals will experience relapse to the contemplation or pre-contemplation stage. Depending on which stage of the model the individual is at, it can be important to provide help or support in order for the individual to progress through the stages. One of the strategies used for this purpose is that of *cognitive* and *behavioural processes*.

• Cognitive and behavioural processes
The stage an individual is at can be ascertained by simple questioning during the screening and lifestyle sessions (see chapter 11). Simply asking the individual which stage they think they are at is sometimes enough, or the answers they give to the instructor's questions can make it evident. Depending on the identified stage of change, the instructor can use strategies known as *cognitive* (experiential) and *behavioural processes* to help the individual, hopefully to arrive at the maintenance stage.

Cognitive processes involve implementing changes to the way individuals think about lifestyle and are divided into five areas (see Table 12.2).

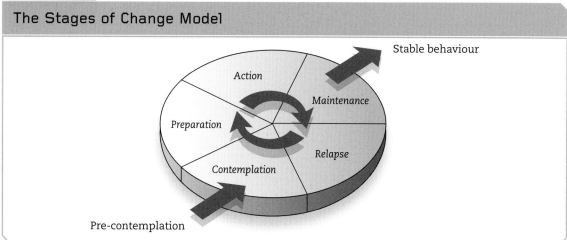

FIG. 12.1

The Stages of Change Model

TABLE 12.1

Description of the stages of change (Prochaska and DiClemente)

Stage	Description
Pre-contemplation (I won't)	The individual does not intend to take any action in the short term (within about six months).
Contemplation (I might)	The individual intends to take action soon but is unsure about the change.
Preparation (I will)	The individual has taken steps towards action and is planning to act, usually within one month.
Action (I am)	The individual has taken action and changed his/her behaviour in the short term.
Maintenance (I have)	Behavioural change has lasted more than six months and the individual is committed to the change.
Relapse	This can happen at any stage and many times over.

NEED TO KNOW
The Stages of Change Model is also known as the *trans-theoretical model*.

NEED TO KNOW
Many professional sports clubs employ psychologists to help implement motivational strategies.

The cognitive processes outlined in Table 12.2 are usually adopted by individuals in the early stages of the Stages of Change Model (pre-contemplation to preparation). Once the individual has moved to the action or maintenance stage, the cognitive processes are not as important as the individual has already thought about the exercise. At this stage, the five *behavioural processes* listed in Table 12.3 can be more important.

Depending on which stage the individual is at, certain cognitive or behavioural processes are more likely to be successful in helping them to move towards the next stage of change. Table 12.4 will guide the instructor to employ the most useful processes at various stages of change.

Even though research is limited in the health and fitness environment in relation to exercise uptake, there is much anecdotal evidence to support the use of the processes. However, instructors should be aware of and focus on the move from the contemplation stage to the action stage, as this is often reported to be the most difficult transition. Instructors should also be aware that many individuals will cite barriers that prevent them from exercising, such as lack of funds, lack of transport, no peer support and self-consciousness, among others. Therefore, it is the role of the instructor to devise strategies and suggest ways for the individual to overcome these potential barriers.

TABLE 12.2

Cognitive processes

Cognitive processes	Description
Consciousness-raising (increasing knowledge)	This relates to seeking new information and understanding, such as ascertaining the benefits of exercise and the risks associated with sedentary behaviour. In terms of health and fitness, examples include visiting one's GP or talking to friends.
Dramatic relief (warning signs)	This relates to the feelings that can be experienced as a result of exercise or sedentary behaviour, such as injury or pain, or tasks becoming more difficult as the individual ages.
Environmental re-evaluation	This involves reflecting on how behaviour can affect other people, such as being a role model and helping others, or sedentary behaviour 'rubbing off' on a friend or partner.
Self re-evaluation	This can be related to re-educating the individual about beliefs related to exercise, such as exercise does not need to be painful to have good benefits, or it can prevent another heart attack.
Social liberation	This relates to helping oneself or others in similar situations and increasing awareness of exercise strategies.

The psychological strategies discussed in this chapter have been shown to influence exercise adherence and, as such, positively impact on the benefits of a healthy lifestyle. As these psychological strategies extend beyond the scope of this book, instructors and individuals are encouraged to increase their knowledge of this particular area as part of self-development and progression. There are many sources available to the instructor (or individual), such as books, websites and courses that relate specifically to the health and fitness industry, in particular to areas such as exercise adherence, performance enhancement, team building, lifestyle management and injury rehabilitation.

 TASK

List the stages of change and explain how various cognitive and behavioural strategies can help individuals to move through the stages.

Motivation

The word 'motivate' is derived from the Latin for 'move' and can be defined as 'the internal mechanisms and external stimuli that arouse and direct our behaviour'. In other words, motivation is what prompts a person to act.

TABLE 12.3

Behavioural processes

Behavioural processes	Description
Self-liberation (understanding the benefits)	This relates to experiencing the benefits of committing to exercise by taking responsibility, which can inspire confidence and self-belief. At this stage the instructor and the individual should make firm resolutions.
Helping relationships	This relates to providing and accepting support for the individual and encouraging empowerment. Buddy systems or personal trainers can be used here. Remind the individual why exercise can be good.
Reinforcement management (rewards)	This involves providing rewards such as T-shirts, badges and certificates for meeting goals and targets, and punishment or forfeits for not.
Counter-conditioning (alternatives)	This involves trying to focus on the positive changes of exercise choices replacing sedentary choices, such as using stairs instead of lifts or walking the dog instead of watching TV.
Stimulus control	This involves trying to remove options for sedentary behaviour, such as hiding the TV remote control, switching on the radio as opposed to the TV and keeping exercise clothes prominent.

This can include the motivation to make lifestyle changes in order to effect weight loss or increase cardiovascular fitness, which relates directly to the cognitive and behavioural processes discussed previously.

In relation to exercise, individuals might have more than one motive to start or maintain an exercise programme, and their motivation could change over a period of time. Many factors can affect motivational preference, so instructors must be aware that they need to regularly address this with the individual. Table 12.5 outlines some of the commonly cited motives for individuals who are either just starting an exercise programme or maintaining an exercise programme.

TYPES OF MOTIVATION

Various motivational factors can influence training in different ways. Athletes may be highly motivated for competition reasons, whereas a beginner may be motivated by factors such as weight loss. These motivational factors may come from external sources, such as a coach or a partner, or from internal factors, such as the individual themselves. These types of

TABLE 12.4

Processes most likely to aid movement towards the next 'stage of change'

Contemplation	Preparation	Action	Maintenance
Consciousness raising: statistics on obesity, information about how exercise can reduce obesity, etc.	Self re-evaluation: small lifestyle changes can have benefits, etc.	Self-liberation: congratulations, you did it and it feels good!	Reinforcement management: well done, you've won a T-shirt for achieving your first goal
Dramatic relief: sedentary behaviour makes you feel lethargic but exercise makes you feel good, etc.	Source materials related to health facts	Post reminders about benefits of exercise, such as weight loss and decreased mortality	Helping relationships: train with a partner – this really helps
Environmental re-evaluation: friends might want to join you, etc.	Research interest from friends and family	Organise buddy groups or sign up to personal training sessions	Counter-conditioning: we have an agreement at work not to use the stairs, etc.
			Stimulus control: my partner only allows the remote after exercise, etc.

motivation are commonly referred to as *extrinsic* and *intrinsic* motivation.

• **Extrinsic motivation** This term is used when individuals are motivated to exercise by external rewards such as certificates, T-shirts, medals and trophies. Many people are motivated extrinsically, so it is prudent to ascertain which extrinsic motivational factors an individual responds best to. However, external rewards can be motivational provided they are not the only reason for taking part in exercise. For adherence

reasons, it is also important to make sure that individuals are not over-reliant on external rewards but focus on internal motivational factors as well.

• **Intrinsic motivation** This term is used when individuals are motivated to exercise by factors such as enjoyment, fun or self-satisfaction. This type of motivation can be linked to outcome goals (see page 199): for example, when an individual achieves a certain exercise goal it could lead to a positive feeling

TABLE 12.5

Common motives for starting/ maintaining an exercise programme

Starting	Maintaining
Health	Enjoyment
Appearance	Role model's influence
Guidance	Variation of activities
Challenge	Social
Submission	Self-esteem
Compulsion	Helping others
Fitness	

5. Keep a reminder in a prominent place (on the individual's desk or fridge door) of the reasons why the individual wants to achieve their specific goals: for example, wanting to increase cardio fitness to run in a charity fun run in six months' time.
6. Introduce the individual to other activities and social events within the exercise facility.
7. Encourage the individual to keep their exercise kit in a prominent place.

TASK
Briefly define the term 'motivation' and list the various extrinsic and intrinsic motivational techniques that are commonly used in the health and fitness industry.

of self-achievement. It might be beneficial to try and identify the type of motivational strategy that might suit the individual during the initial consultation. This can be done by questioning the individual about past exercise history and the success or failure of that exercise history. If a motivational preference cannot be established, try employing motivational techniques, such as those listed below, to assess if they have a positive or negative effect.

COMMON MOTIVATIONAL TECHNIQUES

Below are some common motivational techniques to try with clients.

1. To start with, set short-term goals that are easily achievable.
2. Encourage the individual to find a training partner (use a buddy system).
3. Keep an exercise diary for visual effect.
4. If weight loss is a goal, use pictures of the individual when he or she was slimmer as an incentive to get back to that size.

Goal setting

Goal setting is a simple, yet often misused motivational technique that can provide some structure for an exercise programme. Goals are usually set in order to accomplish a specific task in a specific period of time, such as losing a certain amount of weight for a wedding or being able to run a half marathon within six months. Goal setting can provide a plan of action to help the individual to focus and direct their activities. Information gathered during screening using a template such as the one in Fig. 12.2 can help the instructor and client to set specific goals that are individualised and relevant to that client.

Generally speaking, in relation to exercise there are two categories of goal setting: *process* goals and *outcome* goals. Process goals are goals where the skill is broken down into manageable units for the subject to focus on. Often, form and technique can be classed as process goals as they are task-related rather than results-related. Outcome goals are concerned only with the ultimate outcome – for example, success or failure, winning or losing. In other words, outcome goals are results-related as opposed to task-related. Focus on outcome goals can often affect attention to process goals, which can result in a detrimental effect on the outcome. Therefore, instructors and individuals should try to focus on process goals as well as outcome goals in the initial stages of an exercise programme. Typical process and outcome goals are outlined in Table 12.6.

THE SMARTER PRINCIPLE

Goals in relation to exercise can be set for the short, medium and long term. If only long-term goals were set, the individual might lose interest and exercise adherence could be affected, while achievement of short-term goals could act as a motivational tool for the individual. When agreeing goals with the individual, whether short-, medium- or long-term, the acronym SMART or SMARTER is a useful guide and includes several common characteristics that are often associated with effective goal setting (see Table 12.7).

Regardless of the goals that are set, the instructor and client must review these goals on a regular basis in order to make any changes that are necessary. It is often the case that changes must be made in relation to the lifestyle commitments of the client but changes should also be made if the instructor feels that the client is not 'on-track' to achieve the set goals. Fitness testing is a common method of judging where the client is in terms of their programme. For information on health and fitness testing refer to *Practical Fitness Testing* by Morc Coulson and Dave Archer.

Barriers to achieving goals

One of the main issues an instructor will encounter is ensuring that clients attend regular exercise sessions. This is known as *exercise adherence*. The better the adherence, the greater the chance the clients will achieve their goals. From a health perspective, the more regular exercise is undertaken, the more health benefits will be achieved. There are many reasons that people give for dropping out of an exercise programme or missing exercise sessions. These are otherwise known as *barriers to exercise*. Some barriers, known as *real barriers*, cannot be overcome

TABLE 12.6

Common process and outcome goals	
Process goals	**Outcome goals**
• Be able to do free weight exercises • Be able to run or jog without heart pounding • Establish a routine • Enjoy the exercise • Exercise on your own	• Reduce body fat percentage • Decrease blood pressure • Increase VO_2 max • Complete a marathon • Go down a dress size

for genuine reasons, such as illness and accidents. However, it is possible to overcome some barriers, known as *perceived barriers*, by employing appropriate strategies. Table 12.8 shows examples of perceived barriers and potential solutions to help overcome them. Removing barriers means there is a greater chance of clients adopting and maintaining regular physical activity.

Healthy eating

In terms of goal setting, as well as focusing on activity prescription, many instructors like to give advice or set specific goals relating to nutrition or dietary habits, but it should be stressed that the amount of information should be limited to key areas that follow current

TABLE 12.7

Examples of SMARTER goals

S	Goals must be Specific	If an individual wants to follow a weight-loss programme, be specific about the amount of weight loss that is set as the target. For instance, 0.5kg per week could be a specific target.
M	Training targets should be Measurable	In the example above, 0.5kg per week is a measurable amount, as opposed to 'lose a little weight each week'.
A	Goals should be Adjustable	If an individual finds the target too easy or too hard, the instructor must adapt the programme to suit. In other words, the programme must be adjustable.
R	Goals must be Realistic	Set targets that are achievable: 0.5kg weight loss per week is an achievable target for most people, whereas a target of over 3kg per week might not be achievable by all people.
T	Training targets should be Timebased	For example, 0.5kg weight loss per week can be a short-term target that can lead to an overall loss of about 26kg a year, which is a long-term goal.
E	Goals should be challenging and Exciting	The chances of adherence to the programme are much greater if the programme is exciting in some way.
R	Goals should be Recorded	Make sure that the individual keeps a record of exercise activity as this provides a visual stimulus for the individual and prevents any confusion over a longer term

FIG. 12.2

Goal-setting questionnaire

Client name:	Instructor name:
Stage of change: Preparation	Date:
Client – please write down any goals that you would like to achieve in the...	Agreed goals:
Short term: Take part in aerobics sessions	Process: Enrol in aerobics class twice weekly for first month. Increase to 3 times after that. Design resistance programme 2–3 sessions/week
Medium term: Lose body fat	Outcome: Target loss of 0.5kg/week with mid-term loss of 15kg (ideal weight). Maintain loss at 1-year review
Long term: Maintain the loss	
Client – please write down any barriers to taking part in exercise that you can think of:	Solutions:
Worried about what people think I look like. Difficulty getting to gym	Introduce to buddy (other client in similar position). Possibility of sharing transport

Instructor – identify how you will make the programme SMARTER:
- Specific: weight loss
- Measurable: short- and long-term weight loss target in kg
- Adjustable: increase or decrease based on weekly measurement
- Realistic: in line with current guidelines
- Time based: weekly for the short term leading to a 30-week medium-term goal with maintenance for the longer term
- Exciting: variety often helps
- Recorded: keeping records is key

Instructor – note any potential strategies related to stages of change:
- Include client in goal-setting targets and accompany to gym to book aerobics sessions. Introduce to 'buddy'

TABLE 12.8

Perceived barriers and potential solutions

Perceived barrier	Potential solutions
Time – such as work/family commitments	Design work-based activities. Get client to do family-based activities.
Injury	Depending on the injury, other parts of the body can still be trained and in some situations a non-impact fitness programme such as swimming could be prescribed.
Cost – facility or equipment	Design home or outdoor activities. Any clothing can be adapted. Break down the client perception that they need to follow trends.
Access – getting to facility	Sometimes clients are not even aware of certain facilities. Consider buddy training or working out bus routes. Otherwise, design home-based or outdoor activities.
Age	All fitness levels are relevant. Reinforce the message that exercise can give benefits regardless of age, and stress the importance of reducing the risk of mortality.
Poor self-image	Discourage the client from focusing on 'ideal body types'. Introduce them to like-minded peer groups.
Lack of enjoyment	This could derive from a previous negative experience. Use testimonials to emphasise the fun factor of exercise.

government guidelines. For information or advice beyond these key messages, instructors should refer clients to qualified people such as state-registered dieticians. One of the main sources of information relating to healthy eating is that of the government *Balance of Good Health*, otherwise known as the 'Eatwell Guide', shown in Fig. 12.3. Dietary goals should always be limited to the advice contained within this model.

THE PLATE MODEL

The government has produced this simple visual way of educating the public about a healthy diet.

The Plate Model concentrates on five commonly accepted food groups (rather than individual nutrients) and the proportions of these foods that should be eaten from each group:

FIG. 12.3

The Balance of Good Health Plate Model

- Bread, other cereals and potatoes: for example, bread, cereals, potatoes, rice, noodles, pasta
- Fruit and vegetables: for example, apples, bananas, grapes, kiwi, cabbages, peppers, sweetcorn, peas
- Milk and dairy foods: for example, milk, cheese and yoghurt
- Meat, fish and alternatives: for example, chicken, beef, cod, prawns, eggs, chickpeas, nuts

- Foods containing fat and foods containing sugar: for example, biscuits, jam, margarine, mayonnaise, confectionery, crisps

The intended message is that people should choose a variety of foods from the four largest groups every day. More foods should be eaten from the bread, other cereals and potatoes group and the fruit and vegetables group compared with the milk and dairy foods group and the meat, fish and alternatives group. Foods in

TABLE 12.9

Vitamin uses and effects of deficiency

Vitamin	Main use	Deficiency
Vitamin A (fat soluble)	Retinol – found in plants such as carrots Essential for vision in dim light and is also required for skin, mucous membranes and growth	Night blindness (xerophthalmia)
Vitamin B (water soluble)	B1: Thiamine – release of energy from carbohydrates, especially important for the brain and nerve function B2: Riboflavin – release of energy, especially from protein and fat B3: Niacin – energy release from nutrients B5: Pantothenic acid – utilised in metabolic pathways B6: Pyridoxine – used in many biological reactions; is especially associated with amino acid metabolism B7: Biotin – cell growth and fat metabolism B9: Folic acid – important for protecting the new foetus B12: Cyanocobalamin – important for folate metabolism	Beriberi (nervous system disorder) Problems with lips, tongue, skin Pellagra (skin disorder) Fatigue Skin problems Hair loss, dermatitis Diarrhoea, anaemia Pernicious anaemia
Vitamin C (water soluble)	Ascorbic acid – immune system, aids wound healing and iron absorption	Scurvy (sickness and skin disorders)
Vitamin D (fat soluble)	Calciferol – promotes calcium absorption from food	Rickets (bone softening)
Vitamin E (fat soluble)	Tocopherol – protective effect for cell membranes	Malabsorption of fats, anaemia
Vitamin K (fat soluble)	Menaquinone – especially required to produce blood-clotting proteins	Poor blood clotting, internal bleeding

the smallest group (foods containing fat and containing sugar) should be used sparingly if they are eaten every day or not eaten too often.

FLUID

Water is considered to be the most important nutrient as it makes up between 40 and 70 per cent of total body mass (depending on age, gender and body composition). Many metabolic processes in the body require water to be present, especially digestion and absorption of nutrients and this can be affected if the body becomes too dehydrated. As water is lost through processes such as urination, exhalation and evaporation through the skin, etc., it must be replaced on a daily basis in the form of food (many foods contain water, especially fruits)

TABLE 12.10

Common functions of minerals

Mineral	Common function
Calcium	Used by teeth, bones Muscle and nerve activity Blood clotting
Chloride	Metabolism (the process of turning food into energy)
Copper	Oxygen transportation
Fluorine	Strengthens teeth
Iodine	Thyroid function, metabolism, growth and energy production
Iron	Transports oxygen in red blood cells Protein metabolism
Magnesium	Used in enzyme activity and muscle function Protein building
Manganese	Has a role in the body's anti-oxidant defences
Molybdenum	Involved in the metabolism of DNA
Phosphorus	Present in bones and teeth, a component of all cells
Potassium	Important for brain and nerve function
Selenium	Anti-oxidant, growth and metabolism, pancreas function
Sodium	Regulation of body water content and nerve function
Zinc	Growth and repair, taste perception, anti-oxidant, foetal development

and fluids. The Plate Model does show some fluids, such as milk and fruit juice; however, water, tea and coffee are major contributors to fluid intake (not alcohol). Even though there is no exact recommendation about the amount of total fluid that should be drunk in a day, a general guideline is 6–8 glasses, cups or mugs of fluid.

• **Preventing dehydration** The body loses more water exercising than when at rest, but following simple guidelines can help to prevent dehydration.

- Do not rely on thirst to let you know when you need to drink, as it is an unreliable indicator
- Avoid overdressing as this can cause greater fluid losses; use breathable exercise clothing with wicking capability
- Cut down on your intake of tea/coffee/alcohol; these are all diuretics and cause the body to lose water
- Check the colour of your urine on a regular basis, as this should be pale; a dark yellow/orange indicates possible dehydration

NUTRIENTS

All foods contain chemicals known as nutrients, which are needed for essential processes such as growth and metabolism. Nutrients needed in very small amounts are called micronutrients (vitamins, minerals and fibre) and those that are needed in larger quantities are called macronutrients (proteins, fats and carbohydrates). There are many guidelines in relation to the recommended amounts of macronutrients such as that by the World Health Organization, which suggests an average daily intake (based on the ideal amount of calories) of carbohydrate, fat and protein for the general population should be made up of the following:

- **Fats**: up to 30 per cent (less than 10 per cent from saturated fats)
- **Protein**: 10–15 per cent
- **Carbohydrates**: 55–60 per cent (less than 10 per cent from simple sugars)

All calories should come from macronutrients, which should be balanced (as in the Plate Model) enough in the diet to provide the necessary amounts of micronutrients as well. Vitamins (listed in Table 12.9) are organic substances that are essential in the metabolism of fats, carbohydrates and protein and numerous other functions such as blood clotting, protein synthesis and bone formation.

• **Vitamins** Vitamins are normally categorised into two groups: fat-soluble (transported and stored with lipids) and water-soluble (not stored, transported in water). In most cases, the lack of a vitamin causes severe problems, as shown in Table 12.9.

• **Minerals** There are a number of minerals (inorganic elements) that our bodies must have in order to create specific molecules needed in the body. Table 12.10 lists and describes the common functions of certain minerals. Minerals are often lacking in the diet, which leads to various problems such as osteoporosis through lack of calcium intake and anaemia through lack of iron intake. Other minerals such as sodium are over-consumed by many of the population. A high sodium intake has been linked to hypertension.

ENERGY BALANCE

One of the main concerns resulting from lack of activity is that of overweight and obesity. This

FIG. 12.4

The energy balance equation

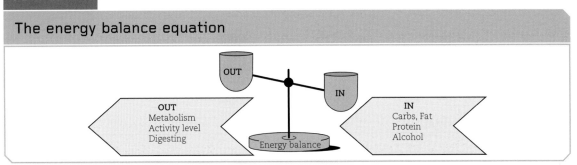

can be explained simply by using something known as the *energy balance equation*. This is used to describe the balance between energy intake (in the form of food) and energy expenditure (in terms of energy stores used for normal function and activity) on a daily basis. Fig. 12.4 shows that if the amount of energy taken in is greater than the amount of energy expended then it is likely that the excess energy will result in weight gain. Conversely, if the amount of energy taken in is less than the amount of energy expended then this could result in weight loss.

EXAMPLE QUESTIONS

12.1 The Stages of Change Model follows what type of pattern?

a) rhythmical

b) cyclical

c) exponential

d) linear

12.2 Approximately what percentage of all individuals will experience relapse back to the contemplation or pre-contemplation stage?

a) 5%

b) 10%

c) 15%

d) 20%

12.3 True or false? Cognitive processes are usually adopted by individuals in the early stages of the Stages of Change Model from not thinking about exercise to the action of taking up exercise.

True   False

12.4 True or false? Behavioural processes are usually adopted by individuals in the later stages of the Stages of Change Model.

True   False

12.5 What is the following a definition of? *'The internal mechanisms and external stimuli that arouse and direct our behaviour'.*

a) cognitive process

b) behavioural process

c) goal setting

d) motivation

12.6 Which term is used to describe when an individual is motivated to exercise by factors such as enjoyment, fun or self-satisfaction?

a) intrinsic motivation

b) extrinsic motivation

c) external motivation

d) behavioural motivation

12.7 When a skill is broken down into manageable units that the subject can focus on, it is otherwise known as what type of goal?

a) SMART

b) outcome

c) process

d) realistic

12.8 The World Health Organization suggests an average daily intake of carbohydrate, fat and protein for the general population should be made up of which of the following?

a) 30% fat, 5–10% protein, 50–55% carbohydrates

b) 30% fat, 10–15% protein, 55–60% carbohydrates

c) 20% fat, 10–15% protein, 60–65% carbohydrates

d) 10% fat, 15–20% protein, 55–60% carbohydrates

12.9 Which of the following vitamins is considered to be important for promoting calcium absorption from food?

a) A

b) K

c) D

d) C

12.10 Which of the following vitamins is considered to be important for producing blood-clotting proteins?

a) A

b) K

c) D

d) C

12.11 Which of the following minerals is considered to be important for brain and nerve function?

a) sodium

b) potassium

c) selenium

d) zinc

12.12 Which of the following minerals is considered to be important for the regulation of body water content and nerve function?

a) sodium

b) potassium

c) selenium

d) zinc

Further reading

American College of Sports Medicine (2017) *ACSM Guidelines to Exercise Testing and Prescription* (10th ed.), Lippincott, Williams & Wilkins

Arthritis Research Campaign (2002) *Arthritis: The big picture*, Arthritis Research Campaign.

Atkinson, R. and Hilgard, E.R. (2014) *Introduction to Psychology* (16th ed.), Wadsworth Publishing

Boutcher, S.H. (2000) 'Cognitive performance, fitness and ageing', in Biddle, S.J.H., Fox, K.R. and Boutcher, S.H., *Physical Activity and Psychological Well-Being*, Routledge, 118–129

British Heart Foundation Health Promotion Research Group (2005) *Coronary Heart Disease Statistics*, Department of Public Health

Bull, S.J., (2000) *Sport Psychology: A self-help*, Crowood

Butler, R.J. (2000) *Sport Psychology in Performance*. Oxford University Press

Coulson, M. and Archer, D. (2009) *Practical Fitness Testing*, Bloomsbury

Cox, R.H. (2011) *Sport Psychology Concepts and Applications* (7th ed.), Brown & Benchmark

Department of Health (2000) *Coronary Heart Disease: National Service Framework for coronary heart disease – modern standards and service models*, Department of Health

Department of Health (2004) *At Least 5 a Week: Evidence on the impact of physical activity and its relationship to health*, Department of Health

Department of Health, Health Survey for England (2007) *Healthy Lifestyles: Knowledge, attitudes and behaviour*, NHS Information Centre for Health and Social Care

Duda, J.L. (1998) *Advances in Sport and Exercise Psychology Measurement*, Fitness Information Technology Inc.

Howley, E.T. and Franks, B.D. (2003) *Health Fitness Instructor's Handbook* (4th ed.) Human Kinetics

Kugler, J., Seelbach, H. and Kruskemper, G.M. (1994) 'Effects of rehabilitation exercise programmes on anxiety and depression in coronary patients: a meta-analysis', *British Journal of Clinical Psychology*, 33: 401–410

McArdle, W.D., Katch, F.I. and Katch, V.L. (2007) *Exercise Physiology* (6th ed.), Lippincott, Williams & Wilkins

NHS Information Centre, Lifestyle Statistics (2009) *Statistics on Obesity, Physical Activity and Diet: England, February 2009*, NHS Information Centre for Health and Social Care

Orlick, T. (1998) *Embracing Your Potential*, Human Kinetics

Prochaska, J.O. and DiClemente, C.C. (1983) 'Stages and Processes of self-change and smoking: toward an integrative model of change'. *Journal of Consulting and Clinical Psychology*, 51(3): 390–395

Van Staa, T.P., Dennison, E.M., Leufkens, H.G. and Cooper, C. (2001) 'Epidemiology of fractures in England and Wales', *Bone*, 29: 517–522

Weinberg, R. and Gould, D. (2014) *Foundations of Sport and Exercise Psychology* (6th ed.), Human Kinetics.

World Health Organization (2002) *The World Health Report 2002. Reducing risks, promoting healthy life*, WHO Press

13 Components and Induction of an Exercise Session

OBJECTIVES

After completing this chapter, you will be able to:

1 List and describe a range of typical baseline health and fitness tests.

2 Explain the term 'induction' in relation to exercise sessions.

3 Describe the process of warm-up, cardio, cool-down, and resistance and flexibility inductions for beginners to exercise.

4 List the common guidelines relating to the use of cardiovascular equipment.

5 List and describe the components of an exercise session.

6 List and describe each of the 'cardio training zones'.

7 Briefly describe the terms 'interval' and 'fartlek' in relation to cardio training.

8 Describe the term 'resistance exercise continuum'.

9 Explain the term 'periodisation' and list its components.

10 List and describe a range of instruction skills.

Introduction

This chapter deals with the components of an exercise session in relation to guidelines within the Professional Standards framework for health and fitness. The chapter also deals with typical baseline health and fitness tests used in the gym environment. Instructors should be able to identify the components of an exercise session and list the guidelines associated with them.

This chapter, along with others in the book, provides information regarding the practical application of theoretical knowledge. This will allow the instructor to design appropriate exercise programmes for apparently healthy individuals, in line with current guidelines for exercise.

Baseline testing

Before an exercise session can be designed and delivered, the instructor should carry out a series of health and fitness tests in order to identify baseline levels for particular parameters. All tests should be explained and agreed by the client and permission must also be given by the client prior to any tests being carried out. It is important that the instructor is aware of potential sources of error associated with each test so that they can take steps to minimise the errors. The main way to minimise errors is to follow a standard testing method known as a *protocol*, which might include pre-test considerations. Once testing has taken place, the results can be compared to certain populations in order to give a categorisation or classification. Population data is known as *normative data* or often referred to as *norm tables*. Instructors should be aware that norm tables can be published that are based on data from specific population groups, such as male, female, obese, deconditioned etc., therefore it is important to make sure the correct tables are used. There are many health and fitness tests available; below is a selection of those useful to the instructor:

BLOOD PRESSURE MEASUREMENT

The instructor should always check that a client's blood pressure (BP) is within normal ranges before starting any programme of exercise. If either of the readings (systolic or diastolic) is in the high (hypertension) range then it is recommended that the test is repeated after a minimum of 10 minutes. If the BP is still high then the instructor should recommend that the test be repeated on a different day before exercise can be commenced. Note: If the BP is still high after a third test then the instructor should advise the client to check with their GP that they are able to undertake a programme of exercise. The only equipment needed for this test is a machine known as a *sphygmomanometer*. Automated versions are reasonably reliable.

• Testing method

1. Subjects should be seated for at least five minutes in a chair with their back supported and their arms bared and supported at heart level. Subjects should refrain from smoking or ingesting caffeine during the 30 minutes preceding the measurement.
2. Wrap the deflated cuff firmly around upper arm at heart level (the bottom edge of the cuff should be approximately 2.5cm (1in) above the elbow crease).
3. Place the cuff over the biceps muscle and fasten it. Make sure it is not too loose.

FIG. 13.1

Blood pressure cuff attachment

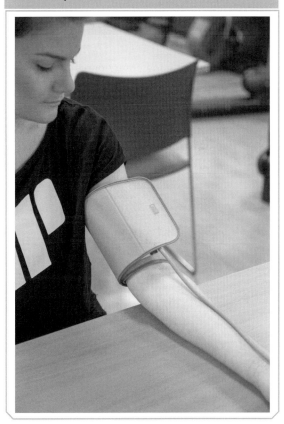

4. The position of the subject's arm and the fastened inflatable pressure cuff can be seen in Fig. 13.1. The arm of the subject should be supported during measurements.
5. Start the machine and record the result.

● **Classification** Ranges for the various stages of blood pressure are shown in Table 13.1. These figures are related to a general adult population.

● **Sources of error** There are many people who become anxious at the thought of having their BP taken. It is important that the client is as relaxed as possible before taking the measurement. One way to do this is to sit the client down and attach the pressure cuff to the upper arm but don't take the reading. Try to distract the client by asking lots of other questions then after about 10 minutes take the reading before the client has time to react. The other main error relates to pre-test conditions. Inform the client not to exercise, eat or drink at least two hours before the test.

BODY MASS INDEX (BMI)

One of the simplest methods of assessing body composition indirectly is body mass index (BMI). The use of body mass index in the general population to indicate obesity is reasonably sound, but in specific groups such as rugby players, it is a poor predictor of body composition. In these groups body mass index is equally affected by gains in lean body mass as it is by fat mass.

● **Analysis** Body mass index can be calculated using the following formula for each individual:

$$BMI = \frac{Weight\ (kg)}{Height^2\ (m^2)}$$

● **Classification** Once the body mass index of a subject has been determined, Table 13.2 can then be used to identify the classification.

TABLE 13.1

Normative values for BP adapted from The National High BP Education Programme 2003	Systolic (mm Hg)	Diastolic (mm Hg)
Hypotension	<90	and <60
Normal	<120	and <80
Pre-hypertension	120–139	or 80–89
Hypertension (stage 1)	140–159	or 90–99
Hypertension (stage 2)	<160	or <100

TABLE 13.2

BMI classifications adapted from the American College of Sports Medicine	
BMI Classifications	**BMI Score**
Underweight	<18.5
Normal	18.5–24.9
Overweight	25–29.9
Class I obese	30–34.9
Class II obese	35–39.9
Class III obese	40 or above

For example, a subject with a body mass index of 26.7 would be categorised as 'overweight' whereas a subject with a body mass index score of 12.5 would be classed as 'underweight'.

- **Sources of error**   The main source of error relates to the equipment being used. Bathroom scales are often inaccurate therefore instructors should avoid letting clients self-test. If using equipment in the gym environment, make sure it is regularly calibrated. Also make sure that repeat measurements are taken at the same time of day if possible to help standardise food and drink intake.

WAIST CIRCUMFERENCE

One of the simplest methods of tracking client weight loss improvement is by measuring waist circumference. The location of fat mass in the body is linked to certain disease. For example, central fat mass (around the waist) is recognised as an independent risk factor for cardiovascular disease. The only equipment needed is a tape measure.

- **Testing method**
1. Subject should stand erect, abdomen and buttocks relaxed, arms at side and feet together.
2. Measure the waist at its narrowest point.
3. Waist circumference is measured midway between the lower rib margin and the iliac crest in the horizontal plane.

- **Classification**   According to the World Health Organization (WHO), a waist circumference of greater than 102cm (40in) for males and 88cm (35in) for females is an indication of an increased risk of developing type II diabetes, coronary heart disease and/or hypertension.

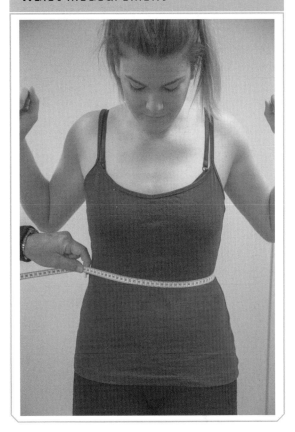

FIG. 13.2

Waist measurement

- **Sources of error**   The main source of error is related to clothing. If taking the measurement over clothes, make sure that the same clothes are used in repeated measurements.

ELECTRICAL IMPEDANCE (BIO-IMPEDANCE)

Bioelectrical impedance is becoming a more frequently used method to assess body composition due to its ease of use, portability and cost. It is based on the principle that the resistance to a current is inversely related to the fat-free mass contained within the body. The fat-free mass contains virtually all the water and electrolytes in the body and hence conducts most of the electric current produced by the bioelectrical device. Fat mass, on the other hand, is very low in water and electrolytes and resists the flow of electric current. There are several machines available on the market. Instructors should follow the procedure related to the particular machine being used. However, the following preparation before testing as recommended by Heyward (1991) should always be followed:

- No eating or drinking in the four hours before the test.
- No exercise for 12 hours before the test.
- Urinate within 30 minutes before the test.
- No alcohol consumption within 48 hours of the test.
- No diuretics within seven days before the test.

Testing method

1 Ensure that the analyser is calibrated before using. This is usually done by comparing the resistance obtained by the analyser to a calibration resistor of known resistance (usually 500W).
2 The subject should lie on a non-conductive surface (if you use a metal bench, ensure that it is covered with blankets and sheets).
3 Legs should be positioned such that the thighs do not touch and hands positioned such that they do not touch the torso.
4 Position the electrodes with reference to the manufacturer's recommendations. This is usually relative to anatomical landmarks such as the ulnar head (Fig. 13.3a) and medial malleolus (Fig. 13.3b) (middle finger and middle toes).
5 The electrode sites should be cleaned to reduce loss of signal and, depending on the type of electrode used, a conducting gel should be placed between the electrodes and the skin.

6 The source electrode produces the current and the reference (detecting) electrode detects it. The drop in voltage between the two reference electrodes determines the impedance.

Classification Once the body fat measurement has been established, Table 13.3 can be used to classify women and men as underweight, overweight or obese.

Sources of error Results using this particular equipment can be affected greatly in the hours leading up to the test, therefore it is extremely important to follow any pre-test guidelines associated with the type of equipment being used. The main error is the hydration status of the client. Instructors should advise the client to keep well hydrated in the days leading up to the test.

SKINFOLDS

Adults carry the majority of fat tissue subcutaneously (under the skin). Skinfold calipers are a simple and inexpensive method of

FIG. 13.3A

Electrode hand connections

FIG. 13.3B

Electrode foot connections

measuring these fat stores. Instructors should be aware that there are certain population groups that this type of testing is not suitable for, such as children and obese individuals. Also, as the test is slightly invasive, the instructor should make sure that the option of a screen is made available. There are many types of caliper available but it is advisable to use metallic calipers if possible.

• Testing method

1. The tester's left hand should raise a skinfold between the thumb and forefinger at the marked site in the required direction, following the natural cleavage lines of the skin (see Fig. 13.4a).
2. There should be slight rolling and pulling action to separate the fold from the muscle beneath.
3. The caliper is held in the right hand and the blades are applied perpendicularly to the fold and 1cm (1/2in) away from the thumb and forefinger (see Fig. 13.4b).
4. Spring pressure is released and value is recorded two seconds later, to the nearest 0.2mm.

TABLE 13.3

Body fat % classifications (adapted from the World Health Organization)

Women				
Age	Underweight	Healthy Range	Overweight	Obese
20–40 yrs	Under 21%	21–33%	33–39%	Over 39%
41–60 yrs	Under 23%	23–35%	35–40%	Over 40%
61–79 yrs	Under 24%	24–36%	36–42%	Over 42%
Men				
Age	Underweight	Healthy Range	Overweight	Obese
20–40 yrs	Under 8%	8–19%	19–25%	Over 25%
41–60 yrs	Under 11%	11–22%	22–27%	Over 27%
61–79 yrs	Under 13%	13–25%	25–30%	Over 30%

5 All skinfolds should be measured three times with a two-second recovery to allow compression of the tissue to return to normal. Measure three times and use the median (middle) value obtained.

• **Classification** There are many normative tables available depending on the method that has been used. Table 13.4 is the table used for the Durnin and Womersley four-site method (measurements taken at four sites). The table predicts body fat percentage relevant to age and the total sum of the skinfolds.

FIG. 13.4A

Grasping a skinfold

FIG. 13.4B

Placement of the caliper

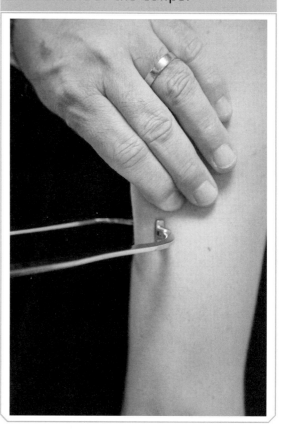

• **Sources of error** Skinfold testing is regarded as quite accurate when the tester is experienced, therefore it is recommended that the instructor practise as often as possible in order to improve their accuracy. It is also advisable to have a more experienced colleague take measurements on the same subjects to check accuracy as well.

SIT AND REACH FLEXIBILITY (ADAPTED)

A common test for flexibility is the *sit and reach test*, whereby an individual sits with straight

TABLE 13.4

Skinfold conversion table (Durnin and Womersley)

	MEN				WOMEN		
	SUM				SUM		
(mm)	16–29	30–49	49+	(mm)	16–29	30–49	49+
20	8.1	12.1	12.5	14	9.4	14.1	17.0
22	9.2	13.2	13.9	16	11.2	15.7	18.6
24	10.2	14.2	15.1	18	12.7	17.1	20.1
26	11.2	15.2	16.3	20	14.1	18.4	21.4
28	12.1	16.1	17.4	22	15.4	19.5	22.6
30	12.9	16.9	18.5	24	16.5	20.6	23.7
35	14.7	18.7	20.8	26	17.6	21.5	24.8
40	16.3	20.3	22.8	28	18.6	22.4	25.7
45	17.7	21.8	24.7	30	19.5	23.3	26.6
50	19.0	23.0	26.3	35	21.6	25.2	28.6
55	20.2	24.2	27.8	40	23.4	26.8	30.3
60	21.2	25.3	29.1	45	25.0	28.3	31.9
65	22.2	26.3	30.4	50	26.5	29.6	33.2
70	23.2	27.2	31.5	55	27.8	30.8	34.6
75	24.0	28.0	32.6	60	29.1	31.9	35.7
80	24.8	28.8	33.7	65	30.2	32.9	36.7
85	25.6	29.6	34.6	70	31.2	33.9	37.7
90	26.3	30.3	35.5	75	32.2	24.7	38.6
95	27.0	31.0	3605	80	33.1	25.6	39.5
100	27.6	31.7	37.3	85	34.0	36.3	40.4
110	28.8	32.9	38.8	90	34.8	37.1	41.1
120	29.9	34.0	40.2	95	35.6	37.8	41.9
130	31.0	35.0	41.5	100	36.3	38.5	42.6
140	31.9	36.0	42.8	110	37.7	39.7	43.9
150	32.8	36.8	43.9	120	39.0	40.8	45.1
160	33.6	37.7	45.0	130	4.02	41.9	46.2
170	34.4	38.5	46.0	140	41.3	42.9	47.3
180	35.2	39.2	47.0	150	42.3	43.8	48.2
190	35.9	39.9	47.9	160	43.2	44.7	49.1
200	36.5	40.6	48.8	170	44.6	45.5	50.0

legs and reaches forwards to record the distance reached with the fingertips using a sit and reach table. Testing usually involves subjects bending forwards as far as possible, which results in a measure of both hamstring and back flexibility. In order to isolate the hamstrings' flexibility measurement from the upper back flexibility measurement, the normal protocol can be adapted as follows.

• Testing method

1. Allow the subject to fully warm up and stretch before the start of the test.
2. The subject's legs should be fully extended with the feet (no shoes) flat against the vertical surface of the box.
3. With one hand placed over the other (palms down, arms straight, fingers outstretched), the subject should sit upright with a normal lumbar curve.
4. The subject should lean forwards as far as possible, sliding his or her hand along the ruler of the sit and reach box while maintaining the normal lumbar curve.
5. The subject should be stopped at the point where the upper back starts to arch or the normal lumbar curve is lost. This point

should be recorded as the *hamstring flexibility score* (Fig. 13.5a).
6. The subject is then allowed to continue to stretch as far as they can. The maximal distance the fingers reach is recorded as the *hamstring/back flexibility score* (Fig. 13.5b).
7. The subject must keep his or hands parallel and should not lead with one hand.
8. Have several attempts and record the best score.

• Classification
There are no separate normative tables available for both hamstring and back flexibility measurements, therefore Tables 13.5a and 13.5b can be used to identify the classification of the combined hamstring and back (maximum score recorded) flexibility score for 16-year-olds and adults.

• Sources of error
The main source of error with this particular test is related to the interpretation of the point at which the tester perceives the transition point between hamstrings and back flexibility. It is advised therefore that the instructor familiarise

FIG. 13.5A

Hamstring flexibility point

FIG. 13.5B

Hamstring/back flexibility point

TABLE 13.5A

Normative table for 16-year-olds (values in cm)

Gender	Excellent	Above average	Average	Below average	Poor
Male	>28	24–28	20–23	17–19	<17
Female	>35	32–35	30–31	25–29	<25

themselves with this test so that they can standardise the way in which they perform it.

HARVARD STEP TEST

This test is designed as a measure of aerobic (cardio) fitness (measured as VO$_2$max). The basis of this test is the assumption that the heart rate response to exercise is directly related to oxygen consumption. Thus, the heart rate response to a fixed-intensity bout of exercise would be lower in a more aerobically fit individual. This is a relatively simple test to administer. However, instructors will need a step of the correct height, a metronome and a heart rate monitor.

- **Testing method**
1. The subject steps on to a bench with one leg, then the other and then steps down in the same manner. Fully extend the legs at the top of the step (see Fig. 13.6).

2. The step rate is set at 22 full steps (up, up, down, down) per minute for women and 24 steps per minute for men.
3. Subjects must maintain this stepping rate for three minutes with the step height always set at 41.3cm (16¼in).
4. After three minutes of stepping the subject remains standing.
5. The heart rate is then taken in bpm.

- **Classification**   Use the formula below to estimate the VO$_2$ max score from the final heart rate achieved by the subject, then use Table 13.7 to determine the classification.

   Men:
   VO$_2$ max (ml.kg^{-1}min^{-1}) = 111.33 – (0.42 x bpm)
   Women:
   VO$_2$ max (ml.kg^{-1}min^{-1}) = 65.81 – (0.1847 x bpm)

- **Sources of error**   This test is simple to administer. However, one of the main limitations

TABLE 13.5B

Normative table for adults (values in cm)

Gender	Excellent	Above average	Average	Below average	Poor
Male	>29	26–28	22–25	19–21	<18
Female	>30	27–29	22–26	19–21	<18

FIG. 13.6

Extended leg during step test

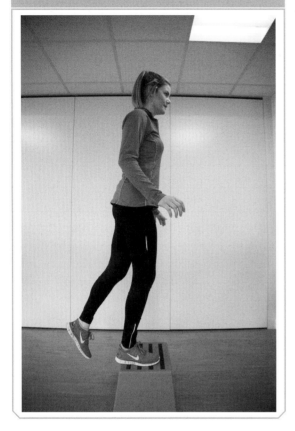

with this test for athletic populations is that the nature of the exercise is not very representative of typical movements in most sports, thus it might be more suitable for a non-athletic population.

COOPER 12-MINUTE RUN

In 1963, Balke developed a test using a 15-minute run to assess aerobic fitness of military personnel. In 1968, Cooper shortened the test to a 12-minute run and adapted it for all populations. The test involves an individual running at their maximal possible pace for a duration of 12 minutes and measuring the total distance covered by the individual. This test is widely used by instructors due to the simplicity of administration of the test and the small amount of equipment that is required. The test can be performed either on a treadmill or on a measured track.

• Testing method

1. Explain the concept of pacing to the subject(s). (Essentially, that they will have to try to maintain their maximum possible pace for 12 minutes).
2. Instruct the subject(s) to cover the longest possible distance in 12 minutes. Walking is permitted, but it is preferable to run.
3. Allow the subject to have a warm-up.
4. The tester starts the stopwatch at exactly the same time as the subject starts the treadmill or sets off.
5. The tester should call out the time at regular intervals.
6. After 11 minutes, the tester should count down the last minute for the subject(s).
7. After 12 minutes, the tester should record the total distance covered by the subject(s).

• Classification
Use the formula below to estimate the VO$_2$ max or use the normative table (Table 13.6) to identify the classification.

$$VO_2 \text{ max} = (d_{12} - 505) / 45$$

Note: In Cooper's formula, d_{12} represents the distance (measured in metres) covered in 12 minutes.

• Sources of error
One of the main limitations of this test is related to something called the *learning effect*. The more times a subject completes the test, the better they will get at choosing the most effective pacing strategy. It is recommended that the instructor allow the client at least two or three attempts on different days for familiarisation purposes.

TABLE 13.6

Normative table for adults (values in metres)

Age	Excellent	Above average	Average	Below average	Poor
Males 20–29	>2800	2400–2800	2200–2399	1600–2199	<1600
Females 20–29	>2700	2200–2700	1800–2199	1500–1799	<1500
Males 30–39	>2700	2300–2700	1900–2299	1500–1999	<1500
Females 30–39	>2500	2000–2500	1700–1999	1400–1699	<1400
Males 40–49	>2500	2100–2500	1700–2099	1400–1699	<1400
Females 40–49	>2300	1900–2300	1500–1899	1200–1499	<1200
Males >50	>2400	2000–2400	1600–1999	1300–1599	<1300
Females >50	>2200	1700–2200	1400–1699	1100–1399	<1100

ROCKPORT FITNESS WALKING TEST

This test is another aerobic fitness test that is based on the time taken to complete a 1-mile (1,609m) walk, finishing heart rate, weight, age and gender. This test provides an option for the instructor who has a client who does not enjoy jogging or running but is quite happy to do a walk test. The test can be performed indoors or outdoors as long as a 1-mile course is measured.

• Testing method

1. Record the weight of the subject.
2. The subject lines up on the starting line.
3. The subject starts walking and the tester starts the stopwatch at the same time.
4. The subject walks 1 mile as fast as possible.
5. Immediately on finishing the walk, record the heart rate (beats per minute) and the time taken.

• Classification
Use the following formula to estimate VO_2 max then use Table 13.7 for the classification:

$$VO_2 \text{ max} = 132.853 - (0.0769 \times BW(kg)) - (0.3877 \times age\ (yrs)) + (6.3150 \times gender) - (3.2649 \times time) - (0.1565 \times HR)$$

Where: Gender = 0 (female) or 1 (male)
Time = walk time to the nearest hundredth of a minute
HR = heart rate (bpm) at the end of the test
BW = bodyweight in kg

• Sources of error
It is quite easy for the client to forget that the point of the test is to walk as fast as possible for the entire mile. It is recommended therefore that the instructor walk with the client in order to motivate them.

• VO_2 max classification
There are many VO_2 max classification tables available for specific age, gender and other such parameters. Table 13.7 shows classifications for general populations related to gender and age.

TABLE 13.7

Male and female normative values for VO$_2$

Female (values in mlO$_2$.kg^{-1}min^{-1})						
Age	V. Poor	Poor	Fair	Good	Excellent	Superior
13–19	<25.0	25.0–30.9	31.0–34.9	35.0–38.9	39.0–41.9	>41.9
20–29	<23.6	23.6–28.9	29.0–32.9	33.0–36.9	37.0–41.0	>41.0
30–39	<22.8	22.8–26.9	27.0–31.4	31.5–35.6	35.7–40.0	>40.0
40–49	<21.0	21.0–24.4	24.5–28.9	29.0–32.8	32.9–36.9	>36.9
50–59	<20.2	20.2–22.7	22.8–26.9	27.0–31.4	31.5–35.7	>35.7
60+	<17.5	17.5–20.1	20.2–24.4	24.5–30.2	30.3–31.4	>31.4
Male (values in mlO$_2$.kg^{-1}min^{-1})						
Age	V. Poor	Poor	Fair	Good	Excellent	Superior
13–19	<35.0	35.0–38.3	38.4–45.1	45.2–50.9	51.0–55.9	>55.9
20–29	<33.0	33.0–36.4	36.5–42.4	42.5–46.4	46.5–52.4	>52.4
30–39	<31.5	31.5–35.4	35.5–40.9	41.0–44.9	45.0–49.4	>49.4
40–49	<30.2	30.2–33.5	33.6–38.9	39.0–43.7	43.8–48.0	>48.0
50–59	<26.1	26.1–30.9	31.0–35.7	35.8–40.9	41.0–45.3	>45.3
60+	<20.5	20.5–26.0	26.1–32.2	32.3–36.4	36.5–44.2	>44.2

GRIP STRENGTH TEST

Grip strength is correlated to many physiological components. For example, grip strength has been shown to correlate to heart disease. Lower grip strength is also associated with reduced health-related quality of life in older men and women and is also considered a useful tool to identify people at risk of mobility limitations, such as difficulty walking or climbing stairs. This is an ideal test that instructors could use for older age clients. A hand-grip dynamometer is the only equipment needed for this test.

• Testing method

1. Ensure the dynamometer is set to zero before use.
2. Adjust the hand grip to suit the subject. Adjust the base and handle until the handle rests on the middle phalange and the base on the first metacarpal.
3. Raise the dynamometer above the head with palms facing inwards.
4. Take a deep breath and squeeze the handle as hard as possible while lowering the arm over a three-second period, elbows fully extended.

5. Record the maximum reading (kg) from three attempts, alternating between the dominant and non-dominant hand.

FIG. 13.7

Hand-grip dynamometer test

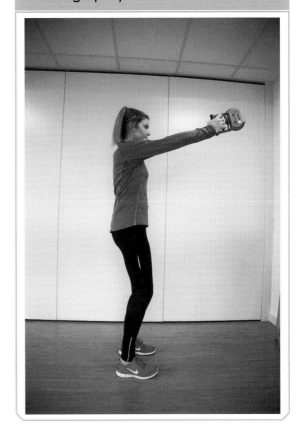

- **Classification** A handgrip strength of 150N (approximately 15kg), equivalent to 20 per cent of bodyweight for a 75kg individual has been suggested as a threshold for the performance of occupational tasks requiring a firm grip. For a 25-year-old male, grip strength of 30kg would be very poor, but the same measurement of 30kg for a 75-year-old male would be average to good. For a classification related to a general population, Table 13.8 can be used.

- **Sources of error** The main error associated with this test is getting the width of the hand grip correct for each client. The instructor should allow the client several attempts using different grip widths while being mindful of fatigue.

PRESS-UP TEST

This is an easy-to-administer test that uses bodyweight rather than an external resistance. The test requires little in the way of equipment and is often used to assess muscular endurance.

- **Testing method**
1. The subject lies on the mat, hands shoulder-width apart, and fully extends the arms (Fig. 13.8a).
2. Lower the body until the elbows reach 90 degrees (mid position), as shown in Fig. 13.8b.
3. Return to the starting position with the arms fully extended.
4. The push-up action is to be continuous with no rest.

TABLE 13.8

Normative values for grip rating

Gender	Excellent	Good	Average	Fair	Poor
Male	>56	51–56	45–50	39–44	<39
Female	>36	31–36	25–30	19–24	<19

FIG. 13.8A

Press-up test start position

FIG. 13.9A

Modified test start position

FIG. 13.8B

Press-up test mid position

FIG. 13.9B

Modified test mid position

5. Record the total number of full-body press-ups completed by the subject before fatigue.

MODIFIED PRESS-UP TEST

It is sometimes the case that individuals are not able to complete full press-ups (or can only do very few) therefore for those who have relatively weak upper body strength, the modified press-

up test can be used. The test is then performed as follows:

• Testing method
1. Lie on the mat, hands shoulder-width apart, bent-knee position & fully extend the arms as in Fig. 13.9a.
2. Lower the upper body till the elbows reach 90 degrees (mid position Fig. 13.9b).

TABLE 13.9A

Normative values for the full-body press-ups

Age	Excellent	Good	Average	Fair	Poor
20–29	>54	45–54	35–44	20–34	<20
30–39	>44	35–44	25–34	15–24	<15
40–49	>39	30–39	20–29	12–19	<12
50–59	>34	25–34	15–24	8–14	<8
60+	>29	20–29	10–19	5–9	<5

3. Return to the starting position with the arms fully extended.
4. The push-up action should be continuous with no rest periods.
5. Record the total number of full-body press-ups completed by the subject before fatigue.

• **Classification** The normative values in tables 13.9a and b are the test standards commonly used to assess press-up performance for both full-body and modified press-ups. These values relate to age.

• **Sources of error** It is important with this test that the instructor is quite strict in what they allow and what they discount as proper form. Fully brief the client before the start of the test so that they are clear about what you will allow.

TABLE 13.9B

Normative values for the modified press-ups

Age	Excellent	Good	Average	Fair	Poor
20–29	>48	34–48	17–33	6–16	<6
30–39	>39	25–39	12–24	4–11	<4
40–49	>34	20–34	8–19	3–7	<3
50–59	>29	15–29	6–14	2–5	<2
60+	>19	5–19	3–4	1–2	<1

Components of an exercise session

Once baseline testing has been completed, a weekly programme of exercise can be designed from which individual sessions can be implemented. A typical exercise session forming part of an overall exercise programme would normally include the following components, as recommended by the American College of Sports Medicine:

1. Warm-up
2. Conditioning phase (including cardio, resistance and flexibility training)
3. Cool-down

Warm-up

Prior to the exercise session, it is essential that the body (and in particular the connective tissues) is fully warmed in order to reduce the potential for injury. Research has shown that perhaps the main factor in muscular injury prevention is muscle temperature (Noonan, 1993): muscle is more elastic when warm and therefore less susceptible to injury.

The entire warm-up should take about 5–10 minutes and should facilitate the transition from rest to the level of exercise required in the main session. The intensity of the warm-up should increase gradually in order to avoid the onset of oxygen debt (see page 94) and can be performed using cardiovascular equipment, such as a treadmill, rower, cycle or step machine or, if no equipment is available, through brisk walking or slow jogging. There is very little difference in the benefits of each method, as they are all capable of stressing the cardiorespiratory system.

The warm-up should aim to achieve a change in a number of physiological responses, in order that the body can work safely and effectively. Typical benefits of a warm-up are:

- An increase in body temperature, specifically core muscle temperature
- An increase in the elasticity of muscular tissues
- A decreased risk of soft-tissue injury
- Activation of the neuromuscular system
- An increase in mental alertness

Conditioning phase

According to the ACSM, the conditioning phase of an exercise session should include one or more of the following types of training: cardiovascular, resistance and flexibility. For a comprehensive session, all areas are recommended.

Cardiovascular training

The cardiovascular session should follow on from the warm-up and can involve the same type of cardiovascular equipment. At the end of the warm-up the heart rate should be at the level required for the cardiovascular session, depending on the goal of the individual. Guidelines for the recommended heart-rate levels and duration and frequency of exercise can be taken from the ACSM guidelines (see chapter 10).

BENEFITS OF CARDIOVASCULAR TRAINING

The main benefits of cardiovascular training, dependent on the intensity, frequency and duration of the exercise, are:

- Weight (fat) loss due to an increase in fat metabolism
- Increased glycogen stores
- Increased aerobic and anaerobic enzymes
- Increase in the number and size of mitochondria
- Increased number of capillaries
- Increased myoglobin levels
- Increased recruitment of muscle fibres
- Increased self-confidence and self-esteem

NEED TO KNOW

For an average individual, it is recommended that energy expenditure per day from exercise should be between 300 and 400 kcal.

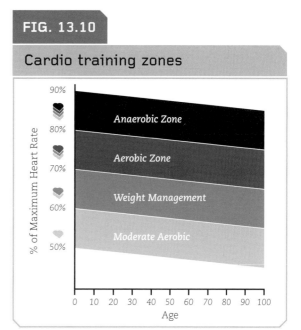

FIG. 13.10

Cardio training zones

Anaerobic Zone

Aerobic Zone

Weight Management

Moderate Aerobic

% of Maximum Heart Rate — 90%, 80%, 70%, 60%, 50%

Age — 0 10 20 30 40 50 60 70 80 90 100

CARDIO TRAINING ZONES

When prescribing cardiovascular exercise, the intensity (how hard the individual should exercise) should be carefully considered. Before agreeing the level of the exercise with an individual, it is useful to understand the benefits of exercising at different levels of intensity, otherwise known as *cardio training zones* (see Fig. 13.10). In basic terms, each specific training zone is related to a heart-rate range in which certain benefits might be expected. The zones are not exact, but they are useful as a guide to cardiovascular training as the benefits relating to each zone are reasonably accurate.

Training zones are based on a percentage window (60–70 per cent, for example) of maximum heart rate (MHR). Within each training zone, subtle physiological effects take place in relation to the heart rate.

• **Moderate aerobic zone: 50–60 per cent MHR** This training zone is mainly suitable for deconditioned individuals,

or individuals who cannot maintain a normal conversation within the heart-rate levels specific to this zone. Regular exercise in this zone will lead to slight improvements in cardiovascular function, depending on the frequency and duration of the exercise undertaken.

Exercise sessions within this zone might only last for a few minutes, so the minimum goal of 20 minutes of cardiovascular exercise, as recommended by the ACSM, should become a target for the client to achieve comfortably before progressing to higher intensity levels such as those in the weight-management zone.

• **Weight-management zone: 60–70 per cent MHR** Training within this zone develops endurance and aerobic capacity, again depending on the frequency and duration of the exercise undertaken. Exercising in this zone also burns fat at a higher rate than the previous zone, which is associated with weight loss. There should also be an

overall improvement in the health status and cardiorespiratory function of the individual.

At this level of intensity, most individuals will be aware of an increase in heart rate, but should be able to carry out a normal conversation. The weight-management zone should be achievable for most beginners to exercise and should be sufficient to bring about overload and hence adaptation to the demands of the exercise. From an exercise adherence perspective, this zone can be beneficial to beginners in that they should feel reasonably comfortable with the level of intensity but should also experience the benefits of adaptation. As the benefits of cardiovascular exercise are affected by frequency, duration and intensity, it is suggested that duration should follow the ACSM guidelines of 20–60 minutes, at a frequency of 3–5 days per week. In terms of intensity, a greater amount of energy will be expended at 70 per cent of maximum heart rate compared to that expended at 60 per cent for the same amount of time; this will affect the overall amount of fat used as fuel for the exercise.

• Aerobic zone: 70–80 per cent

MHR This zone is sometimes referred to as the 'fitness' zone and can also be described as the moderate-to-vigorous intensity zone. The ability of the body to transport oxygen to and carbon dioxide away from the working muscles can be developed and improved by training in this zone. At this level of intensity breathing rate is increased, so this level is more appropriate for individuals who are used to exercising on a regular basis. Some individuals will still be able to carry out a conversation at this level, but others might find it difficult to do so while still maintaining regular breathing.

• Anaerobic zone: 80–90 per cent

MHR Training in this zone can help to develop the lactic acid system (see chapter 6). In this zone the individual's anaerobic threshold is

normally reached. The amount of fat utilised (in percentage terms) as the main source of energy in this zone is greatly reduced, as glycogen stored in the muscle is the predominant source of fuel. One of the by-products of using glycogen as a fuel is lactic acid. The body can normally remove and deal with low levels of lactic acid, but as levels of lactic acid start to increase the body reaches a point at which it can no longer remove the lactic acid from the working muscles quickly enough. This happens at a heart rate, and hence intensity, that is specific to each individual and is usually accompanied by a rapid rise in heart rate and a slowing of intensity. This point is known as the *onset of blood lactate* or *OBLA*. The correct type of training can increase the body's ability to remove lactic acid for a longer period of time, thus delaying the OBLA. Due to the high-intensity levels associated with this zone, it is mainly suitable for athletes or those individuals who have a considerable base of fitness. It is important to note that at higher intensity levels such as these, the risk of orthopaedic injuries and cardiac complications is increased.

DURATION OF CARDIOVASCULAR TRAINING

Regardless of the training zone being used, the guidelines for cardiovascular endurance as stated by the ACSM suggest a duration of 20–60 minutes continuous or intermittent exercise (intermittent meaning an accumulation of 10-minute bouts of exercise throughout the day). A distinction should be made between this definition and intermittent types of cardiovascular training that are sometimes used by individuals as a training method. Two common types of intermittent cardiovascular training are *fartlek* and *interval training*.

• **Fartlek** The term *fartlek* loosely translates as 'speed play' and involves alternating the

intensity level throughout the duration of the cardiovascular session. This kind of training appears to be random in relation to recovery periods and intensity levels. Typical training is conducted at around 70 per cent of VO_2 max with bursts of higher intensity, around 85–90 per cent of VO_2 max.

● **Interval training** Interval training is a more systematic form of training that uses precise work:recovery ratios. For example, an individual will maintain a constant speed for a certain period of time at an aerobic level, then increase the intensity to an anaerobic level for a short period of time. The intensity will then be reduced to a lower level than at the start to allow the individual to recover. The process then begins again.

There is a complex interaction between the exact levels of aerobic and anaerobic intensity and the period of recovery, and a number of sessions are normally required in order to fine-tune this. Fig. 13.11 provides an example of one cycle in an interval training session and can be explained as follows:

- A–B: This is the individual's normal level of aerobic intensity.
- B–C: The intensity is gradually increased to an anaerobic level.
- C–D: The anaerobic level is maintained for a short period of time.
- D–E: The level is quickly lowered in order to recover.
- E–F: The intensity is increased to the starting level.
- F: The process repeats itself.

Because of the high-intensity levels associated with interval and fartlek training, a higher degree of physical stress is placed on the structures of the body, especially at the joints. It is advisable for an individual to have an adequate cardiovascular base of fitness before

FIG. 13.11

Example of an interval training session

undertaking this type of exercise. As all of the energy systems in the body are used during this type of training (see chapter 6), careful planning is needed to target the systems so that the individual can achieve his or her goals. The following points should be considered:

- The current fitness level of the individual
- The fitness goals of the individual
- The energy systems applicable to the goals identified
- The duration and intensity of the build-up to the required level
- The duration and intensity of recovery periods
- The duration and intensity of the normal work periods
- The number of repetitions of each cycle (overall duration)

High Intensity Interval Training (HIIT) has increased in popularity in the health and fitness industry. There is no specific formula for HIIT as high-intensity training has been around in one form or another for centuries. Training programmes designed by coaches or instructors often mimic the work-to-rest ratios that are typical of the specific sport or event. The work-to-rest ratio is dependent on many factors, including the experience of the individual and the goal of the training programme. General guidelines for work-to-rest ratio can be related to the intensity or HIIT zone as shown in Table 13.10.

However, before those individuals new to HIIT undertake a programme of this type of exercise it is recommended that certain guidelines or procedures should be adhered to. For example, instructors should make sure that individuals establish a good level of cardio fitness before progressing to HIIT. Individuals should also begin with the maximum recommended rest period specific to the intensity of the exercise performed and should gradually reduce the rest period as they become accustomed to the training.

NEED TO KNOW

It has been shown that there are many benefits of regular HIIT such as weight loss, improved cardio fitness and improved insulin resistance. It should be emphasised, however, that there are risks involved in exercises at almost maximal heart rate levels.

COOL-DOWN FOLLOWING A CARDIOVASCULAR WORKOUT

The *cool-down* is sometimes referred to as a *warm-down* and these two terms can be used interchangeably. Due to the increased heart rate of the cardiovascular part of the session, individuals need to take time to gradually reduce the heart rate and blood pressure to near resting levels. This is known as the cool-down.

The ACSM recommends a period of approximately 5–10 minutes for this part of the exercise session. Individuals can use the same type of cardiovascular equipment used in the warm-up and cardiovascular endurance sessions to achieve this, but at a level that gradually reduces in intensity. In general terms, the cool-down should help to:

- Disperse lactic acid
- Prevent blood pooling
- Return the body systems to normal levels
- Assist in maintaining venous return
- Reduce the potential for hypotension and dizziness
- Help to dissipate body heat

NEED TO KNOW

As a general guide, the intensity levels of the exercise should be reduced gradually throughout the cool-down until the heart rate is below 100 bpm.

TABLE 13.10

Typical HIIT ratios

Intensity (HIIT zone)	Work-to-rest ratio	Work duration	Rest duration
95–100%	1:3	Up to 10 seconds	15–30 seconds
85–90%	1:2	10–45 seconds	0.5–1.5 mins
75–85%	1:1	45 secs–2 mins	1.5–2 mins

• Cool-down guidelines

- Reduce the level of intensity gradually
- Elicit feedback from participants on the level of intensity
- Be in a position to observe all participants
- Stretches can be included on the move if the client is balanced

Resistance training

Resistance training can be performed using different forms of exercise, such as resistance machines, free weights and bodyweight exercises. Depending on the facility, a large range of resistance machines and free weights will be available. Prior to working with clients at a new facility, instructors should familiarise themselves with the machines when working at a new facility. The resistance training part of the session should start with a warm-up and finish with a cool-down.

BENEFITS OF RESISTANCE TRAINING

Many benefits are associated with resistance training, depending on the intensity of the resistance, the number of sets and repetitions performed, the rest periods and many other variables. Common benefits include:

- Reduced risk of osteoporosis
- Increase in muscle mass
- Increase in bone mass
- Increase in glucose tolerance
- Increased joint integrity
- Reduced back pain
- Improved posture
- Reduction of hypertension
- Reduced risk of diabetes
- Increased strength of connective tissue

Regardless of the goal of the resistance training element of the session, the instructor should be aware of the *overload principle*. This simply states that in order for any strength gains to occur (known as a *training response*), the client must exercise at an intensity greater than normal. In relation to weight training this can come about by manipulating either the weight used, the number of sets performed or the frequency of the training. One of the easiest ways to help the client self-monitor progression is to establish the correct weight for the chosen *repetition maximum* (discussed later in this chapter) then instruct the client that when they can do two repetitions more than originally prescribed then they should increase the weight by a small amount.

WARM-UP FOR RESISTANCE TRAINING

It is not advisable to perform any muscular contractions against a resistance until the muscle or muscle groups have been prepared. This can be done by performing a number of contractions using a lighter weight than prescribed for each resistance exercise in the programme.

MAIN ACTIVITY

Prior to designing an exercise programme that includes resistance training, it is necessary to establish the number of repetitions to be performed during the training session. This can be done either during the individual's induction or during the first training session. For example, if an individual decides to perform 10 repetitions, he or she needs to find a weight that they can lift successfully 10 times but fail on the 11th repetition. If the individual can perform more than 10 repetitions easily, the weight should be increased; if the individual cannot perform 10 repetitions, the weight should be decreased. This is a trial and error method that becomes easier to administer as the instructor gains experience.

• The resistance exercise continuum

Common goals for a resistance training programme include muscular strength, endurance, hypertrophy and power. Training programmes are normally devised in relation to the specific goal, but can differ depending on the level of knowledge and experience of the individual. Although there is no such thing as an optimum programme for muscular strength, endurance, hypertrophy or power gains due to the many variables that can affect the nature of a resistance training programme, there is a general and commonly used guide that shows the intensity required to elicit specific gains. This is known as the *resistance exercise continuum* (see Fig. 13.12).

Adapted from Baechle, 2016. (Increasing darkness of colour and increasing font size correspond to increased adaptation for the relevant goal at the repetition maximum.)

In simple terms, to elicit strength gains it is logical to train with heavy loads, so the number of repetitions performed will be low. If, on the other hand, muscular endurance is the goal, it is logical to train with lighter loads and therefore perform a higher number of repetitions.

FIG. 13.12

The resistance exercise continuum

Depending on the outcome goal (strength, endurance, power or hypertrophy), a certain range of repetitions is recommended to elicit the appropriate adaptation, as can be seen in Fig. 13.12. This range is not exact and there is a certain degree of overlap due to the many variables that can affect adaptation to the specific training. The amount of weight (intensity) to be used can be based on a percentage of the individual's 1RM. As an alternative, Tables 13.11, 13.12 and 13.13 provide a guide to training for strength, endurance and power/hypertrophy.

TABLE 13.11

Strength training recommendations for novice, intermediate and advanced			
	Novice	Intermediate	Advanced
Intensity (% of max)	50–60	60–80	80–100
Sets	1–2	2–3	2–5
Reps	10–15	8–12	1–8
Frequency (sessions per week)	1–2	2–3	3–5
Rest (minutes)	1.5	2	3

TABLE 13.12

General endurance training recommendations

	Short-term	Medium-term	Long-term
Reps	12–25	25–50	50–100
Sets	3	2–3	1–2
Rest	30–60 secs	1–1.5 mins	1.5–2 mins
Method	Light weights	Bands, med balls, etc.	Bodyweight

NEED TO KNOW
Research has found little difference, in terms of adaptation, between single-set and multiple-set resistance training programmes.

FREE WEIGHTS VS. RESISTANCE MACHINES

One of the current anecdotal debates within the health and fitness industry is whether to advocate free weight exercises, resistance machine exercises or both. Resistance machines vary greatly between manufacturers with respect to ergonomic design, range of adjustment and planes of movement, so it is impossible to advocate one method of resistance training over another. The advantages and disadvantages of both resistance machines and free weights must be taken into account on an individual basis (see Table 13.14). It is the instructor's responsibility to advise individuals of the benefits of both methods of resistance training and to take into account the individual's preference before designing an exercise programme.

• **Structure of the resistance training session** Regardless of whether resistance machines, free weights or both are incorporated

TABLE 13.13

General power/hypertrophy training recommendations

	Set 1	Set 2	Set 3
Intensity (% of 1RM)	70	60	50
Reps	4–6	6–8	8–10
Rest (minutes)	2–2.5	3	3.5

TABLE 13.14

Advantages and disadvantages of different types of resistance training

	Advantages	Disadvantages
Free weights	Many exercises can be performed with limited equipment Uses synergists and fixators in a functional isotonic way Full range of motion is available Less expensive compared to machines Relatively portable	More instruction required for safety and correct technique Often require a training partner for safety purposes Do not always appeal to a broad range of users
Resistance machines	Relatively easy to learn and therefore to instruct The weight selected does not need to be calculated The weight setting can be changed easily	The plane of motion is set by the machine, which is not functional Can sometimes limit range of motion Seated positions do not replicate most functional movements Seat supports negate the use of core stabilisers Lack of synergist and fixator use Relatively expensive compared to free weights

into a training programme, within each training session the larger muscle groups should be exercised before the smaller muscle groups. This is to prevent the smaller muscle groups becoming fatigued and affecting the exercises in which they assist the larger muscle groups. For example, if the triceps muscles were exercised to fatigue before the bench press was performed, the individual would achieve a lower than normal weight, as the triceps muscles assist the pectorals in this exercise.

COOL-DOWN FOLLOWING RESISTANCE TRAINING

The requirements of a cool-down following resistance training are similar to those following cardiovascular training. At the end of each exercise, the individual should perform several repetitions of the same exercise using a lighter weight than that used in the main activity.

TASK

List the components of an exercise session and briefly outline the ACSM recommendations relating to each component.

RECOVERY

One of the most overlooked aspects of resistance training is that of recovery. It is essential that enough time is given for muscle tissue to repair and rebuild after exercise. As a general guideline, a period of no less than 24 hours should be allowed between training sessions for the same muscle groups and in some cases, such as a particularly intense session, a period of 48 hours would be more appropriate. The instructor could advise the client of several potential strategies that might aid recovery such as:

- Maintain regular sleep patterns
- Keep well hydrated at all times
- Try to maintain a healthy diet
- Avoid alcohol as much as possible
- Use active recovery rather than just stop
- Employ static stretching post-exercise
- Try ice baths

Flexibility training

Flexibility is the range of possible movement in a joint. Flexibility exercises can be performed prior to the main cardio session after the warm-up or at the end of the cool-down, depending on preference. The ACSM guidelines for stretching do not state when the exercises should be carried out, only that they should be performed a specific number of times per week at a certain intensity (2–4 reps of 10–30 seconds). If stretches are performed prior to the conditioning phase,

they are known as *pre-stretches*, and if they are performed after the conditioning phase, they are known as *post-stretches*. The actual stretches performed are the same; it is just the name that is different.

The stretching exercises included within each exercise session should be related to the specific muscle groups that are going to be or were used during the session. Many stretches are in use throughout the health and fitness industry and the type of stretch employed can depend on several factors, including the preference of the instructor who is designing the exercise programme. However, certain stretches can place unnecessary strain on particular joints. These stretches are known as *contraindicated* stretches and should be avoided. Table 13.15 describes some typical stretches used in the health and fitness industry. For the purpose of this book, however, the focus will be upon stretches that are not considered to be contraindicated.

As with the other components of health-related physical fitness, it is essential that the instructor performs the correct technique when demonstrating any stretches in order for the client to copy.

Periodisation

The term *periodisation* is used in both sport and health and fitness. It relates to programme design and the process of manipulation of a programme of exercise at regular intervals, known as cycles. Although periodisation is used predominantly by athletes in order to organise their training programmes so that they 'peak' at competition times, it is also used in the health and fitness industry as a goal-setting tool: the regular manipulation of an exercise programme is thought to elicit optimal gains in one or more of the components of fitness.

TABLE 13.15

Typical stretches

Muscles stretched	Key points	Demonstration
Pectoralis major Anterior deltoid	1. Stand with your feet hip-width apart 2. Clasp your hands behind your back 3. Straighten your arms 4. Raise your arms until you feel tension 5. Maintain neutral spine	
Trapezius Latissimus dorsi Posterior deltoid Biceps brachii	1. Stand with your feet hip-width apart 2. Clasp your hands in front of you 3. Straighten your arms away from your body 4. Separate the scapula by pushing your shoulders forward	

TABLE 13.15 (CONTINUED)

Typical stretches

Muscles stretched	Key points	Demonstration
Triceps	1. Stand with your feet hip-width apart 2. Raise one elbow above your head 3. Reach towards the opposite scapula 4. Increase the stretch by pushing your elbow with the opposite hand	
Hip flexors	1. Adopt the lunge position 2. Lower the hips forward and down 3. Keep your body upright 4. Keep your front foot flat	

TABLE 13.15 (CONTINUED)

Typical stretches

Muscles stretched	Key points	Demonstration
Quadriceps	1. Clasp the front of your foot 2. Take your heel towards your bottom 3. Keep your knees almost together 4. Maintain neutral spine	
Hamstrings	1. Sit on the floor with neutral spine 2. Place the heel of one foot on the inside of the opposite knee 3. Lean forward from the waist 4. Maintain neutral spine	

TABLE 13.15 (CONTINUED)

Typical stretches

Muscles stretched	Key points	Demonstration
Hip adductors	1. Sit on the floor with your knees apart and the soles of your feet together 2. Place the forearms on the inside of the lower leg as shown in the picture 3. Apply pressure to the legs until you feel tension 4. Maintain a neutral spine	
Hip abductors	1. Sit on the floor with one leg out straight in front of you 2. Cross the opposite leg over the straight leg 3. Sit upright and hug your knee to your chest	

In order to achieve this, it is common to monitor ongoing performance so that the programme can be adjusted accordingly depending on the nature of the results. The programme can be organised into intervals known as cycles. Each type of cycle has a different time allocation:

- Microcycle: this is the shortest period of training within an exercise programme and normally refers to the number of training sessions in a seven-day period (that is, short-term planning). Obviously, any goals within such a short period of time need to be achievable in relation to the individual.
- Mesocycle: this is a repeating series of microcycles over a period of several weeks (that is, medium-term planning). The goals in a mesocycle should be achievable yet flexible, as they can be manipulated following analysis of the microcycles within it.
- Macrocycle: this is a series of mesocycles, normally over a period of a few months to several years (that is, long-term planning). Information gathered from microcycles and mesocycles can be used to confirm or readjust the long-term goals of the macrocycle.

Each microcycle contributes to the goals of the mesocycles, which in turn will contribute to the goals of the overall macrocycle. It is important that the instructor constantly revises the goals of each cycle due to the constant interaction of one cycle on another. Planning a programme of exercise using periodised cycles can be useful as it can give individual short-, medium- and long-term goals (see chapter 12). This has been shown to have a positive effect on adherence to exercise, not only for beginners but for regular exercisers as well. When designing an exercise programme, it is recommended that it is recorded simply and accurately, so that the individual can use it as a reference during

exercise sessions. There are many ways of designing a periodised exercise programme but one of the more common methods is that of the step-loading model.

THE STEP-LOADING METHOD

Simple progressive overload training programmes known as *linear periodisation* are the most commonly used training method for those new to exercise in which variables such as training intensity (weight used) and volume (repetitions x sets) are manipulated. Although this is a good way to develop a strength foundation, the training can be boring and repetitive for the individual, as well as leading to staleness and increasing the risk of repetitive loading injuries. The opposite is the case with the step-loading programmes, which are thought to decrease the risk of repetitive injuries. Step-loading models normally include 2 or 3 short cycles (microcycles) of increases in intensity followed by a short cycle of decreased intensity (similar in intensity to the second cycle) before repeating the process again. The simple model shown in Fig. 13.13 can relate to either cardiovascular or resistance training programmes.

It can be seen in the example of a step-loading model that short cycles of specific intensities can be performed in sequence.

FIG. 13.13

Typical step-loading model for cardio or resistance training

Cycles

Again, the intensities are just examples, which depend on many variables relating to the individual and the event that they are training for. The step-loading model can also be thought of in terms of low-, moderate- and high-intensity cycles that increase in intensity when repeated. Quite often these cycles are a week long, where the moderate-training intensity week is usually representative of an average training week and the low and high-intensity weeks are adjusted to this level. There are many types of periodisation models available but the instructor should bear in mind that for most health and fitness clients, variety of exercises is key to avoiding staleness and improving adherence.

FIG. 13.14

Example session plan template

SESSION PLAN:	Number:			Page:	
Instructor name:	Client name:			Ability level:	
Objectives:					

Duration (reps, seconds, circuits, etc.)	Exercises (name muscles used and draw diagrams, where needed)	Equipment	Sets	Intensity (speed, rpm, weight, level)	Alternative and progression (and coaching points)

First aid point:

Tel:

Resources:

Music:

Recording exercise programmes

There are many ways of recording exercise programmes, but for a session within a microcycle it is common to use a session card (see Fig. 13.14) that provides information relating to one session only. A typical session card contains all the information relevant to the individual performing the exercise, as well as information regarding the specific exercise plan. Be aware that information contained on a session card can be confidential so must be treated as such.

Induction sessions

The term *induction* is used to describe the process of the instructor explaining to the client the details and requirements of the exercise session in relation to their specific programme, and showing them how the exercise session will be carried out in the environment they are going to use. For example, inductions that take place in a gym aim to familiarise the client with the operation of the equipment and the performance of the exercises in relation to the session. Therefore, as well as explaining how to operate any equipment, the induction should take the client through each component of the exercise session in turn (warm-up, cardio, cool-down, resistance and flexibility) to make sure they understand and practise each component. This will also give the instructor the opportunity to identify client training intensities in relation to cardiovascular and resistance equipment settings.

Client induction sessions are normally carried out following a successful client screening session (see chapter 11) in which it was agreed that the client could begin a programme of exercise. There are no specific guidelines relating to client induction procedures, which is one of the reasons why all health and fitness facilities tend to have their own methods for client induction. However, regardless of the method used for induction sessions, common guidelines can be applied. These guidelines relate to a client induction for the cardiovascular, resistance and flexibility components of the session to be performed.

WARM-UP, CARDIO AND COOL-DOWN INDUCTION

The facility in which the instructor is working will determine the type of cardiovascular machines available. When working at a new facility, instructors are advised to familiarise themselves with the machines prior to inducting individuals.

Before individuals begin a programme of exercise, they need to be given an induction relating to their specific exercise programme, starting with the first session. Following an explanation of the controls of the cardiovascular machines, it is usual for the instructor to take the individual through their training session in order to establish cardiovascular intensity levels for the warm-up, main activity and cool-down. There are many methods of inducting individuals on cardiovascular machines depending on the individual instructor's preference. However, in order to be consistent in the delivery, it is advisable to use a logical approach such as the acronym IDEA, which can be used regardless of the cardiovascular machine being used:

I   Introduce the exercise
D   Demonstrate the correct technique
E   Explain the exercise using minimal coaching points
A   Activity: observe the client doing the activity on the machine

It is important that instructors use correct technique when demonstrating so that the individual does not copy 'bad' technique. As the visual demonstration will provide a great deal of information for the individual, the verbal information that supplements this can be kept to a minimum. When the individual is using the machine, the instructor should maintain a dialogue in order to give them relevant information on performance and technique. The instructor should then aim to identify the suitable training intensity.

Even though a vast range of cardiovascular training equipment is available, there are many common guidelines that can be employed when using the equipment (see chapter 15).

The treadmill can be used for both walking and running, but is associated with greater impact on the joints than other cardiovascular machines. The cycle doesn't involve any impact, so can be used for individuals who need to reduce the amount of impact to the joints, such as those with obesity or arthritis. As with the treadmill, the cycle can be used for either aerobic or anaerobic conditioning, depending on the intensity of the exercise. Stepping and rowing are also non-impact machines that can be used for individuals wishing to avoid any impact on the joints, but it is important to remember that rowing can place a greater amount of stress on the lower back than other methods of cardiovascular exercise.

It is also recommended that information regarding health and safety is given to the individual during the induction session. Fire exits and emergency procedures can be pointed out, as well as water and toilet facilities. The individual should also be made aware that they should terminate exercise at any time should they feel unwell or unable to continue.

NEED TO KNOW

The loss of balance that sometimes occurs when a treadmill comes to a stop is due to confusion in the brain, as the brain is used to objects in the distance becoming nearer when moving forward.

RESISTANCE INDUCTION

Most beginners to resistance training are unfamiliar with the operation of resistance machines and free weights. It is therefore important to give clear explanations of how to operate resistance machines and the techniques involved in resistance training before the individual begins an exercise programme.

As with the cardio induction, the instructor usually takes the individual through their resistance training session in order to establish intensity levels for the warm-up, main activity and cool-down. There are many methods of inducting individuals in relation to resistance training, depending on the individual instructor's preference. However, in order to be consistent in the delivery, it is advisable to use a logical approach such as the NAMSIT method:

N   Name the machine or exercise
A   Area of the body working
M   Muscle group name
S   Silent demonstration
I   Instruct client to try
T   Teach the client

This approach can be used regardless of the resistance machine being used. It is important that instructors use good technique when demonstrating to prevent the individual copying 'bad' technique.

As with the cardiovascular demonstration, the visual demonstration for resistance exercises will provide a lot of information, so supplementary verbal information should be kept to a minimum.

When the individual is using the machine, the instructor should maintain a dialogue in order to give relevant information on performance and technique. The instructor should then aim to identify the suitable training intensity required for each resistance exercise.

FLEXIBILITY INDUCTION

As with any other part of the induction it is important that the instructor provides a technically correct demonstration of all the stretches included in the exercise programme. The gym environment should have a matted area for stretching. It is logical to start with standing stretches and then progress to seated stretches, in order to decrease the heart rate progressively. Once the instructor has demonstrated the stretch, the individual should perform it. The instructor should then give feedback about the individual's technique and give instructions about the intensity and duration of the stretch.

TASK
Explain the two common methods of cardiovascular and resistance training induction, referring to their acronyms.

Instruction skills

There are many skills that an instructor can have in relation to the delivery of an induction session and exercise sessions to follow. Communication, observation, feedback and reflective practice are considered to be some of the main skills that should be developed.

COMMUNICATION

When communicating with a client, verbal (with an emphasis on speaking), para-verbal (through voice tone and stress on words) and non-verbal (by the use of gestures) methods are all equally as important. If communicating verbally, it is advised to keep the amount of information to a minimum due to the limited capacity of short-term memory. For this reason, instructions should be kept simple and clear. As over 70 per cent of communication is achieved through non-verbal means it is more effective to demonstrate the required exercise technique rather than use verbal commands. Although not an easy thing to do, it is recommended to keep all demonstrations silent. Any verbal communication can then be limited to the main points relating to safety.

OBSERVATION

During any induction session the instructor needs to observe the client at all times. When observing, the instructor should keep in mind aspects of safety, performance, reinforcement and correction.

- **Safety**   There are many potential hazards and dangers in a gym environment, therefore the instructor needs to be aware of their position in relation to the client at all times. For example, the instructor should be able to see the face of the client at all times so that they can monitor for signs of any undue distress.

- **Performance**   Instructors should constantly monitor the performance of a client. Facial expressions and appearance can often indicate the intensity level of the particular exercise.

- **Reinforcement** Reinforcing correct movement can be used as a motivational tool. Clients will often feel better about themselves when they are told their performance is good.

- **Correction** It is important to correct client technique as soon as possible. Demonstrations can be repeated or the *mirroring technique* could be used. This is where the instructor positions themselves in front of the client and performs the technique required at the same time as the client so that they can follow.

FEEDBACK

Giving feedback to the client can take place both during the induction and afterwards. It is important that feedback should be given in a positive manner but, during the performance, should be limited to minor correction points and regular praise, which helps the client's motivation. At the end of the session, feedback can be more explicit and linked to the client's goals.

Reflective practice

As with any profession, it is good practice to implement strategies that help improve personal performance and development. One method that is commonly employed to do this is called *reflective practice*. There is a great deal of research relating to reflective practice. However, in practical terms it can be thought of as a period of consideration following delivery of a session in order to identify what went well and what didn't, possible reasons why, and what could be done to improve the next session. There are many different types of reflective models available to the instructor; however, the use of a post-session assessment form (see Fig. 13.15), which is completed by the instructor and a colleague, is a simple and effective way to help improve performance.

This requires a colleague (preferably more experienced) to observe a particular session, so the permission of the client would need to be sought before the session is observed. The colleague should be made aware of the assessment form used prior to the session so that they are familiar with the process. During the session, the observer should indicate with a tick in column A if, in their opinion, each criteria was met effectively. At the end of the session, the instructor could do the same by judging their own performance. Any difference in opinion could be identified at the foot of the assessment form, which could then be discussed between the colleague and instructor. It is crucial that the instructor then tries to devise an action plan (taking into account the views of the colleague) in order to address the issues that were identified.

FIG. 13.15

Session delivery assessment form

SESSION DELIVERY ASSESSMENT FORM

Client:	Date:	A = Colleague B = Instructor	A	B
Prepare and teach an individualised exercise session				
1		Meet clients punctually and make them feel at ease	✓	✓
2		Collect any new information from clients about response to previous activity	✓	✓
3		Discuss the objectives and exercises that you have planned for the session and how these link to clients' goals	✓	✓
4		Discuss the physical and technical demands of the planned exercises and how clients can progress or regress these to meet their goals	✗	✓
5		Assess, agree and review clients' state of readiness and motivation to take part in the planned exercises	✓	✓
6		Negotiate, agree and record with clients any changes to the planned exercises that will meet their goals and preferences and enable them to maintain progress	✓	✓
Teach and adapt planned exercises				
7		Use teaching and motivational styles that are appropriate to clients and accepted good practice	✓	✓
8		Provide clients with an appropriate warm-up	✓	✓
9		Make best use of the environment in which clients are exercising	✓	✓
10		Provide instructions, explanations and demonstrations that are technically correct, safe and effective	✓	✓
11		Check clients' understanding of instructions, explanations and demonstrations	✓	✓
12		Adapt verbal and non-verbal communication methods to make sure clients understand what is required	✗	✓

FIG. 13.15 (CONTINUED)

Session delivery assessment form

13	Ensure clients can carry out the exercises safely on their own	✓	✓
14	Observe and analyse clients' performance, providing positive reinforcement throughout	✓	✓
15	Correct techniques at appropriate points	✓	✓
16	Progress or regress exercises according to clients' performance	✓	✓

Bring exercise sessions to an end

17	Allow sufficient time for the closing phase of the session	✓	✓
18	End the exercises using a cool-down that is safe and effective for clients	✓	✓
19	Provide clients with positive reinforcement about their performance	✗	✓
20	Give clients your feedback on the session	✓	✓
21	Explain to clients how their progress links to short-, medium- and long-term goals	✓	✓
22	Discuss other possible activities with your clients	✓	✓
23	Leave the environment in a condition suitable for future use	✓	✓

Difference criteria numbers = 4, 12, 19

Plan of action strategies:

1. Forgot to discuss demands of exercise session. Use a checklist in future.

2. Could have used non-verbal cues at times to reinforce technique. Try to do this in next session for all exercises.

3. Negative feedback needs to be given along with positive.

EXAMPLE QUESTIONS

13.1 According to research, what is considered to be the main factor in muscular injury prevention?

a) strength

b) muscle temperature

c) flexibility

d) stretching

13.2 In terms of cardiovascular training at the end of the warm-up, the heart rate should be at what level?

a) the heart rate is irrelevant as long as the individual is warm

b) 60% max heart rate

c) that required for the cardiovascular session to follow

d) maximum

13.3 In relation to cardio training zones, what range of heart range maximum is the 'weight management zone'?

a) 50–60%

b) 60–70%

c) 70–80%

d) 80–90%

13.4 In relation to cardio training zones, what range of heart range maximum is the 'aerobic zone'?

a) 50–60%

b) 60–70%

c) 70–80%

d) 80–90%

13.5 Which of the following are considered to be the main benefits of cardiovascular training?

a) decreased fat metabolism, increased glycogen stores, increased aerobic and anaerobic enzymes, increased number and size of mitochondria

b) increased fat metabolism, decreased glycogen stores, increased aerobic and anaerobic enzymes, increased number and size of mitochondria

c) increased fat metabolism, increased glycogen stores, decreased aerobic and anaerobic enzymes, increased number and size of mitochondria

d) increased fat metabolism, increased glycogen stores, increased aerobic and anaerobic enzymes, increased number and size of mitochondria

13.6 What type of training is otherwise known as 'speed play'?

    a) interval

    b) continuous

    c) intermittent

    d) fartlek

13.7 Which cycle of periodisation is usually associated with a seven-day period?

    a) minicycle

    b) microcycle

    c) mesocycle

    d) macrocycle

13.8 Which cycle of periodisation is usually associated with a period of a few weeks?

    a) minicycle

    b) microcycle

    c) mesocycle

    d) macrocycle

13.9 Which cycle of periodisation is usually associated with a 12-month period?

    a) minicycle

    b) microcycle

    c) mesocycle

    d) macrocycle

13.10 The ACSM guidelines for stretching suggest holding the stretch for what period of time?

    a) 5–10 seconds

    b) 15–30 seconds

    c) 10–20 seconds

    d) 30–45 seconds

13.11 The acronym IDEA refers to what?

    a) induction for cardiovascular machines

    b) induction for resistance machines

    c) the screening process

    d) risk stratification

13.12 Which of the following cardiovascular machines is normally associated with higher impact?

    a) cycle

    b) stepper

    c) treadmill

    d) rower

Further reading

American College of Sports Medicine (2017) *ACSM Guidelines to Exercise Testing and Prescription* (10th ed.), Lippincott, Williams & Wilkins

Baechle, R.T. (2016) *Essentials of Strength Training and Conditioning* (4th ed.), Human Kinetics

Bompa, T.O. (2009) *Periodisation Theory and Methodology of Training* (5th ed.), Human Kinetics

Bouchard, C., Blair, N.S., and Haskell, W. (2012) *Physical Activity, Fitness and Health* (2nd ed.), Human Kinetics

Howley, E.T. and Franks, B.D. (2003) *Health Fitness Instructor's Handbook* (4th ed.), Human Kinetics

Marieb, E.N. (2011) *Human Anatomy and Physiology* (11th ed.), Benjamin Cummings Publishing Company Inc.

McArdle, W.D., Katch, F.I. and Katch, V.L. (2007) *Exercise Physiology* (6th ed.), Lippincott, Williams & Wilkins

Noonan, T.J., Best, T.M., Seaber, A.V. and Garrett, W.E. (1993) 'Thermal effects on skeletal muscle tensile behaviour', *American Journal of Sports Medicine*, 21(4): 517–522

Ross, J.S. and Wilson, J.W. (2018) *Anatomy and Physiology in Health and Illness* (13th ed.), Churchill Livingstone

Sewell, D., Watkins, P. and Griffin, M. (2012) *Sport and Exercise Science: An Introduction* (2nd ed.), Hodder Arnold

Stratton, G., Jones, M., Fox, K.R., Tolfrey, K., Harris, J., Maffulli, N., Lee, M. and Frostick, S.P. (2004) 'BASES position statement on guidelines for resistance exercise in young people', *Journal of Sports Sciences*, 22(4): 383–390

Tortora, G.J. and Grabowski, S.R. (2017) *Principles of Anatomy and Physiology* (15th ed.), Wiley

Kenney, L., Wilmore, J.H. and Costhill, D.L. (2019) *Physiology of Sport and Exercise* (7th ed.), Human Kinetics

14 Monitoring Exercise Intensity

OBJECTIVES

After completing this chapter, you will be able to:

1 List and describe the cardiovascular training zones associated with the health and fitness industry.

2 Explain the various methods of monitoring cardiovascular and resistance exercise intensity.

3 Calculate percentages of heart rate maximum.

4 Explain the term 'over-training' and list the typical signs.

Introduction

This chapter deals with common methods of prescribing and monitoring exercise intensity employed within the health and fitness industry in relation to guidelines within the Professional Standards for health and fitness. Instructors should be able to list the common methods of monitoring cardiovascular and resistance exercise intensity and explain each within the context of the health and fitness industry.

Other chapters in the book provide information regarding the practical application of the theoretical content which, along with the information covered in this chapter, will provide instructors with the understanding and ability to design appropriate exercise programmes for apparently healthy individuals, in line with current guidelines for exercise.

Exercise intensity

Intensity refers to the difficulty level of a particular exercise or, in simple terms, how hard the exercise feels to the individual. When designing an exercise programme, instructors can prescribe intensity levels that best suit the individual's goals. For example, an individual might have weight loss and toning as goals. In this case, the instructor could set cardiovascular intensity within the weight-management training zone and resistance training intensity at around 10–12 RM (see chapter 10).

Monitoring the intensity level at which an individual is exercising can also help instructors to adjust the exercise programme accordingly. Monitoring can give the instructor information regarding fitness progression or any drop in performance that might indicate signs of over-training, allowing him or her to use this information to make necessary adjustments to the programme.

When prescribing exercise at a specific intensity, it is useful to understand the physiology in relation to each component of fitness (see chapter 10). Intensity levels of both cardiovascular exercise and resistance exercise can be monitored in several different ways. Monitoring intensity within a health and fitness environment is not as accurate as monitoring within a laboratory environment, but is still useful if the lack of accuracy is taken into consideration.

Monitoring cardiovascular intensity

Several methods can be used to prescribe and monitor a particular cardiovascular exercise intensity for an individual, including heart rate, metabolic equivalents, self-perception (rate of perceived exertion) and communication skills (the talk test).

HEART RATE

One of the most common methods of prescribing or monitoring cardiovascular intensity is the heart rate method. As the intensity of the exercise increases, the heart rate of the individual increases in a linear fashion. It therefore follows that, as training zones are related to a percentage of maximum heart rate, the percentage of maximum heart rate that has been agreed for the exercise can be related to the goals of the individual. For example, if the individual wants to develop aerobic fitness, he or she should exercise at a heart rate level of 70–80 per cent of their maximum (the aerobic zone). This can be written as 70–80%HRM.

Two steps need to be taken in order to convert the chosen percentage of heart rate maximum into beats per minute. First, the maximum heart rate of the individual needs to be found; second, the required percentage of this maximum needs to be calculated.

• Step 1: Calculating the maximum heart rate of an individual
Maximum heart rate can be calculated by using one of two methods: one way is to carry out a maximum graded heart rate test, and the other is to use a formula for predicting maximum heart rate.

Maximum graded heart rate test
Several tests are available in which intensity is increased until the point at which there is no rise in heart rate, even though the intensity is continuing to increase. This type of test is reasonably accurate, but is not suitable for any individual who is tested within the health and fitness environment, as National Occupational Standards guidelines recommend that instructors advise exercise intensity only up to a maximum of 90 per cent of heart rate maximum.

Predicted maximum heart rate
As an alternative to a maximum graded heart rate test, the following formula can be used to predict maximum heart rate:

Maximum Heart Rate = 220 – age

For example, a 23-year-old person would have a predicted maximum heart rate of 197 bpm (220 – 23 = 197) and a 45-year-old person would have a predicted maximum heart rate of 175 bpm (220 – 45). Even though there are errors associated with this method of estimating maximum heart rate (there can be an error of plus or minus 12 bpm using this method), it is commonly used and is suitable for the health and fitness industry. Other prediction equations are available, such as that by Tanaka, Monahan and Seals (2001) for healthy men and women:

Maximum Heart Rate = 208 – (0.7 × age)

There is also the equation by Miller (1992) for less fit individuals:

Maximum Heart Rate = 217 – (0.85 × age)

● **Step 2: Calculating the percentage of the maximum heart rate in bpm** Once the maximum heart rate has been established, it is possible to calculate the percentage of heart rate maximum that is required for the individual in beats per minute (bpm): the maximum heart rate for the individual is multiplied by the chosen percentage. For instance, a 32-year-old individual

TABLE 14.1	
Metabolic equivalents for various activities	
Activities between 3 and 6 METs	**Activities of more than 6 METs**
Housework: Polishing Cleaning windows Making beds Mopping floors Vacuuming Hanging washing Sweeping Gardening – light work **Activities:** Slow walking Brisk walking Slow cycling Slow swimming Skating Gentle aerobics Yoga Dancing (ballroom, etc.) Golf Table tennis **Sports:** Fencing Archery Cricket	**Housework:** Any heavy housework Any heavy gardening **Activities:** Jogging Running Brisk cycling Brisk swimming Wheeling in wheelchair High-impact aerobics Martial arts Circuit training Skipping **Sports:** Dancing Tennis Horse riding Squash Basketball Football Gymnastics Fencing Skiing Rugby Netball Boxing

needs to perform the exercise at 70–80 per cent of maximum heart rate (the aerobic zone). The instructor should calculate the individual's training intensity heart rates at 70 and 80 per cent of maximum as follows:

1. Predicted maximum heart rate for the individual is 220 – age (32) = 188 bpm
2. 70 per cent of maximum (188 bpm) = 188/100 × 70 = 131 bpm
3. 80 per cent of maximum (188 bpm) = 188/100 × 80 = 150 bpm

Note: Round the answer to the nearest whole number.

Therefore, in order to exercise at the desired intensity, the individual would need to keep his or her heart rate between 131 bpm and 150 bpm. Over a period of time, if the individual could maintain this heart rate but at an increased speed, this would indicate that the individual was becoming fitter. This is one method of monitoring cardiovascular fitness.

METABOLIC EQUIVALENTS (METS)

The intensity of an exercise can be linked to the amount of energy expended by the individual: the greater the intensity level of the exercise, the greater the energy expenditure required to sustain that level. A *metabolic equivalent* or *MET* is a way of expressing expenditure in either calories (kcal) or volume of oxygen (VO_2). The resting value of 1 MET is expressed as follows:

$$1 \text{ MET} = 3.5 \text{ mlO}_2.\text{kg}^{-1}\text{min}^{-1} \text{ or } 1\text{kcal.kg}^{-1}\text{hr}^{-1}$$

It follows that an exercise that requires four times as much energy than that used at rest would have a value of 4 METs and an exercise that requires 10 times as much would have a value of 10 METs, and so on. Even though MET values are commonly shown on cardiovascular machines, the use of metabolic equivalents seems to be restricted to medical

use for exercise prescription. If the machines used do not display MET values, there are many published tables that estimate them for a range of activities (see Table 14.1). These activities can extend to household chores and outdoor activities as well as fitness facility activities.

Note: This table has been adapted from a variety of sources and should be used as an approximation of metabolic equivalent values related to various activities.

As METs have a value expressed in calories, if the weight of the individual is known, then the amount of calories expended during a particular exercise can also be calculated. Take, for example, a 75kg person exercising at 10 METs for one hour:

10 METs = 10 kcals per kilo of bodyweight every hour, and 10 (kcals) × 75 (kg) = 750. Therefore, this person would expend 750 kcals.

NEED TO KNOW
Any activities between 3 and 6 METs are considered moderate-intensity physical activity. Any activities greater than 6 METs are considered vigorous-intensity physical activity.

RATE OF PERCEIVED EXERTION (RPE)

Another method of setting and monitoring the appropriate exercise intensity for an individual is to use the *rate of perceived exertion (RPE) scale* (see Table 14.2), which was first introduced by Dr Gunnar Borg and is sometimes known as the Borg Scale.

The RPE scale is a method of measuring the subjective feelings of an individual during exercise. The individual's perception of the level of difficulty during cardiovascular exercise has been found to correlate very strongly with heart rate. For this reason, the RPE scale is widely used as an alternative to heart rate.

Two different scales are commonly used: the 6–20 scale and the revised 0–10+ scale, also known as the *category ratio* or *CR-10 scale*. The individual is shown the scale during exercise and asked how he or she feels compared to the words on the scale. This perception is then used to estimate either the percentage of heart rate maximum or the heart rate. For example, if the individual states that the exercise feels 'somewhat hard', this equates to level 13 on the 6–20 scale, which corresponds to approximately 130 bpm or 70 per cent of

TABLE 14.2

Rate of perceived exertion (Borg) scale

6–20 scale	0–10 scale	Estimate of %MHR
6	0 Nothing at all	
7 Very, very light	0.3	
8	0.5 Extremely weak	50%
9 Very light	0.7	55%
10	1 Very weak	60%
11 Fairly light	1.5	65%
12	2 Weak	70%
13 Somewhat hard	2.5	75%
14	3 Moderate	80%
15 Hard	4	85%
16	5 Strong	88%
17 Very hard	6	92%
18	7 Very strong	96%
19 Very, very hard	8	98%
20	9	100%
	10 Extremely strong	
	11 Absolute maximum	

Adapted from *ACSM Guidelines for Exercise Testing and Prescription*, Lippincott, Williams & Wilkins (2017).

MHR. Depending on the goals of the individual, the instructor can recommend an RPE level at which to exercise without the need to monitor heart rate.

Even though the subjective perception of exercise intensity correlates well with heart rate, it is important to note that various individuals carrying out exactly the same exercise session might report different levels of RPE. There are many factors that could affect this perception rating, such as fitness levels, exercise familiarity and illness.

NEED TO KNOW

Research has shown that perception rating on the 6–20 scale correlates closely with heart rate: for example, a 'very light' rating equates to 9 on the scale, which would be a heart rate of approximately 90 bpm.

TALK TEST

Although the talk test is not a particularly scientific method of determining cardiovascular exercise intensity, it can be used as an alternative to heart rate, METs or RPE due to the ease of administration. The talk test is simply a matter of talking to the individual during exercise and gauging the level of intensity from the response of the individual. If the individual is able to carry out a normal conversation, this usually indicates that he or she is in either the weight-management zone or the lower end of the aerobic zone.

If the individual becomes breathless and has difficulty maintaining a normal conversation, this usually means he or she is in the anaerobic zone. The instructor can then adjust the level of intensity accordingly, depending on the goal of the exercise session.

Once the required level of intensity of a cardiovascular exercise session has been attained using the talk test method, the instructor can empower the individual to take responsibility for maintaining that level in subsequent exercise sessions. The individual should be informed that they can progress by increasing the intensity of the exercise, as long as they are still able to carry out a normal conversation.

TASK

List the methods of monitoring cardiovascular intensity and briefly describe how each method is used.

Monitoring resistance intensity

When prescribing the intensity of a resistance exercise (how heavy the weight should be), the instructor can use a percentage of the maximum capability of that individual, known as 1 repetition maximum or 1RM. However, one disadvantage of this method is that the maximum capability of the individual must be found before a percentage of this can be calculated. As the individual would have to perform to maximum capability, the risk of injury would be high and not in line with recommended guidelines.

An easier method would be to use a multiple of the repetition maximum, such as 10RM or 15RM, which means the maximum weight the individual can lift 10 or 15 times respectively. The ACSM guidelines for strength and endurance are given in multiples of RM. For example, in order to gain strength it is recommended that an individual performs resistance exercise using weights within the range of 8–12RM, and to improve endurance using weights within the

TABLE 14.3

Repetition maximum compared to percentage of maximum capability

Repetition maximum	% of maximum capability
1	100.0
2	93.5
3	91.0
4	88.5
5	86.0
6	83.5
7	81.0
8	78.5
9	76.0

Adapted from Baechle (2016).

range of 10–15RM. Research has shown that the multiple of repetition maximum correlates to a percentage of the maximum capability (see Table 14.3).

CALCULATING REPETITION MAXIMUM

When trying to establish the amount of weight an individual can lift for a specific number of repetitions (repetition maximum), a certain procedure should be used to ensure that the individual is sufficiently warmed in order to minimise the risk of injury. If the instructor and the individual have agreed that an intensity of 12RM is going to be used for a particular exercise, the individual should first perform 12 repetitions of a known light weight. Then add more weight depending on the ease of the first set and have the individual perform another 12 repetitions. Repeat this process until the individual can perform 12 repetitions only, and not 13. Ensure

that sufficient rest is given between sets to recover: two to three minutes should be sufficient. The final weight (or load) that the individual could lift 12 times (but fail on the 13th) is the 12RM for that particular exercise. This process should then be repeated for all of the exercises in the resistance training programme.

For progression purposes (and assuming that the multiple repetition maximum chosen is to remain constant), when the individual is capable of comfortably performing the chosen repetition maximum, the weight can be increased by a small amount. If the individual cannot perform the number of chosen repetitions at the increased weight, he or she must revert to the original weight. This type of in-built progression is easy to implement and, as such, the instructor should empower the individual to take control of monitoring their own progression.

TASK

Briefly describe the term *repetition maximum* and explain how it is used to determine the intensity of the resistance exercise to be performed.

Over-training

One of the problems associated with the inability to monitor exercise intensity correctly is the potential for *over-training*. The term 'over-training' is generally considered to relate to a physiological and psychological state brought about by an excessive amount of training over a long period of time. There is also a term *over-reaching,* which is related to occurrence in the short term. In other words, over-reaching can lead to over-training if it is not dealt with effectively. It is generally thought that over-training is mainly linked to athletes but it is

TABLE 14.4

Typical signs of over-training

Symptom category	Symptom indication
Movement/coordination	• Increased incidence of rhythm/movement problems • Lack of prolonged concentration • Reduced ability to correct movement errors
Condition	• Decrease in endurance, strength, speed, etc • Increased resting heart rate • Menstrual disruptions, rapid weight loss, persistent colds • Insomnia, headaches, DOMs. • Tries to deviate from set programme
Psychological	• Increased non-typical behaviour • Anxiety, depression, lacks motivation • Increased introvert behaviour • Negative attitude; gives up easily • Can't cope with difficult situations such as competition

also prevalent within the health and fitness industry. Although it is difficult to diagnose and not without contention, there are typical signs of over-training, such as those in Table 14.4, that the instructor should be aware of. If the instructor suspects that over-training might be an issue, the training load of the client should be reduced until such time as the instructor feels the client has fully recovered.

Monitoring for over-training is difficult as there is no foolproof testing method available. There are, however, two methods that are commonly used: resting heart rate profiling and mood state monitoring using questionnaires such as the Profile of Mood States (POMs) questionnaire. Resting heart rate profiling essentially involves monitoring a client's resting heart rate on a daily basis. Trainers would often associate any sustained increase over a period of a few days with a need to decrease training levels. The POMs questionnaire was originally developed as a psychological tool and has been adapted for sports and health and fitness environments to assess the mood of clients. Baseline testing is performed to create a mood 'profile' of the client, which is then repeated on regular occasions. Deviations from the baseline profile are sometimes thought to indicate potential over-training.

EXAMPLE QUESTIONS

14.1 What is the formula for predicted maximum heart rate?

a) 200 – age

b) 210 – age

c) 220 – age

d) 230 – age

14.2 True or false? Predicted maximum heart rate can have an error of up to plus or minus 12 beats per minute.

True   False

14.3 True or false? A graded maximum heart rate test should be used on all individuals to find their maximum heart rate.

True   False

14.4 What is the predicted maximum heart rate for a 29-year-old person?

a) 201 bpm

b) 191 bpm

c) 189 bpm

d) 199 bpm

14.5 What is 70% of predicted maximum heart rate for a 40-year-old person?

a) 106 bpm

b) 116 bpm

c) 126 bpm

d) 136 bpm

14.6 What is 80% of predicted maximum heart rate for a 20-year-old person?

a) 160 bpm

b) 170 bpm

c) 150 bpm

d) 180 bpm

14.7 What is 55% of predicted maximum heart rate for a 31-year-old person (round up)?

a) 101 bpm

b) 124 bpm

    c) 114 bpm

    d) 104 bpm

14.8 What is the equivalent value of 2 MET?

    a) 3.5 $mlO_2.kg^{-1}min^{-1}$

    b) 5 $mlO_2.kg^{-1}min^{-1}$

    c) 7 $mlO_2.kg^{-1}min^{-1}$

    d) 9.5 $mlO_2.kg^{-1}min^{-1}$

14.9 What is the equivalent value of 1 MET?

    a) 1.0 $kcal.kg^{-1}hr^{-1}$

    b) 1.5 $kcal.kg^{-1}hr^{-1}$

    c) 2.0 $kcal.kg^{-1}hr^{-1}$

    d) 2.5 $kcal.kg^{-1}hr^{-1}$

14.10 How many kilocalories would an 80kg person expend in 30 minutes doing an exercise valued at 5 METs?

    a) 100

    b) 200

    c) 300

    d) 400

14.11 How many kilocalories would a 60kg person expend in 2 hours and 30 minutes doing an exercise valued at 4 METs?

    a) 400

    b) 500

    c) 600

    d) 700

14.12 Which of the following statements is most accurate in regards to the definition of 12RM?

    a) A weight that can be easily lifted 12 times

    b) A weight at which the performer fails on the 12th repetition

    c) A weight that can be lifted at least 12 times

    d) A weight that can be lifted 12 times and not 13 times

Further reading

American College of Sports Medicine (2017) *ACSM Guidelines to Exercise Testing and Prescription* (10th ed.), Lippincott, Williams & Wilkins

Baechle, R.T. (2016) *Essentials of Strength Training and Conditioning* (4th ed.), Human Kinetics

Bouchard, C., Blair, N.S., and Haskell, W. (2012) *Physical Activity, Fitness and Health* (2nd ed.), Human Kinetics

Howley, E.T. and Franks, B.D. (2003) *Health Fitness Instructor's Handbook* (4th ed.), Human Kinetics

Marieb, E.N. (2011) *Human Anatomy and Physiology* (11th ed.), Benjamin Cummings Publishing Company Inc.

McArdle, W.D., Katch, F.I. and Katch, V.L. (2007) *Exercise Physiology* (6th ed.), Lippincott, Williams & Wilkins

Miller, W.C., Wallace, J.P. and Eggert, K.E. (1992) 'Predicting max HR and the HR-VO$_2$ relationship for exercise prescription in obesity' from *Medicine and Science in Sports and Exercise*, 25(9): 1077–1081

Ross, J.S. and Wilson, J.W. (2018) *Anatomy and Physiology in Health and Illness* (13th ed.), Churchill Livingstone

Sewell, D., Watkins, P. and Griffin, M. (2012) *Sport and Exercise Science: An Introduction* (2nd ed.), Hodder Arnold

Tanaka, H., Monahan, K.D., and Seals, D.R. (2001) 'Age predicted maximal heart rate revisited' from *Journal of American College of Cardiology*, 37(1): 153–156

Tortora, G.J. and Grabowski, S.R. (2017) *Principles of Anatomy and Physiology* (15th ed.), Wiley

Kenney, L., Wilmore, J.H. and Costhill, D.L. (2019) *Physiology of Sport and Exercise* (7th ed.), Human Kinetics

15

Free-weight, Resistance Machine and Cardio Exercises

OBJECTIVES

After completing this chapter, the reader should be able to:

1   List and describe common cardio, free weight and resistance machine exercises associated with the health and fitness industry.

2   Describe how each exercise is carried out in terms of technique.

3   List the major muscles and synergists responsible for the exercises.

4   Give alternatives for each exercise.

5   Explain the logical and scientific rationale for avoiding particular exercise techniques.

Introduction

This chapter deals with common cardio, free weight and resistance machine exercises employed within the health and fitness industry. Within the Professional Standards framework, instructors should be able to list the common resistance exercises and the major muscles used in each. Instructors should also be able to describe how to perform and give alternatives to each exercise. The chapter also deals with exercise techniques that could increase risk of musculoskeletal injury.

This chapter builds upon the information in other chapters of this book, regarding the practical application of the theoretical content,

to provide the instructor with an understanding of the correct performance technique associated with a range of free weight, cardio and resistance machine exercises.

Free-weight and resistance exercises

The choice of performing resistance exercises using free weights or machines is an individual preference. However, there are several issues that are common within the health and fitness environment (see Table 15.1).

TABLE 15.1

Health and fitness issues

Issue	Comment
Type of equipment	**Barbell** A long bar with weights attached at either end for use with both hands. **Dumbbell** A small bar with weights attached at either end for use with one hand only. **Collars** These are used on barbells and dumbbells to prevent the weights coming off. They must be used at all times with free weights. **Benches** Make sure benches are robust enough to use with free weights. **Floor mats** These are recommended in the area where free weights are used, to prevent damage to the floor and the weights.
Speed of execution	All exercises must be performed under control so that muscles are worked through their full range and posture is not compromised.
Range of movement	Always use the full range of movement possible for each exercise. Try to keep the repetitions continuous rather than resting at either the start or mid-point.
Breathing	A breath out is normally done prior to the exertion of the exercise. If this is confusing, just breathe normally.
Alignment	Neutral posture must be maintained during all exercises.
Storage	Return free weights to their storage racks after use.
Handling technique	When lifting free weights from the floor, adopt a squat position and keep the weights close to the body.
Levers	To increase the intensity of the exercise, take weights further from the body (increase lever length).
Gravity	For free weights to be effective the weight must travel in a vertical direction.

The examples of free weight and resistance machine exercises given in this chapter are typical of those used by beginners to this type of training. There are many other exercises common to the health and fitness environment, which can be considered to be more advanced, or for those with at least several months' experience of weight training. It is crucial that all beginners to resistance exercises are shown the correct technique in a demonstration prior to performing the exercise themselves. Beginners must also be shown safety-related points, such as how to attach collars to weight lifting bars, how to pick up and return free weights from their storage racks and how to keep the exercise area clear of obstructions. As research is sparse in relation to musculoskeletal injury as a consequence of resistance training, the following examples describe how to perform each exercise with what is considered to be safe technique within the health and fitness industry. The major and synergist muscles for each exercise are also listed, along with alternatives for each exercise that involve the same muscle groups.

EXERCISE 15

(a) and (b): Chest Press

Major muscles used: Pectoralis major

Synergist muscles used: Anterior deltoid, triceps, serratus anterior

- Main movement: Horizontal adduction of the shoulder/extension of the elbow
- Make sure the feet are placed firmly on the ground and that the upper arms are parallel to the floor.
- The palms should be facing forwards and the hands should be directly above the elbows.
- Raise the weights in an arcing motion, keeping them in line with the chest until the arms are fully extended.

Awareness points: Keep the hands directly above the elbows at all times and make sure that the wrists remain firm. Lower the weights under control until the upper arms are parallel with the floor. Maintain a normal lumbar curve at all times.

Safety point: Starting the movement with the upper arms parallel to the floor should ensure that the pectoralis major is responsible for the majority of the effort. Starting at a lower point could strain the anterior deltoid as this muscle will then be taking most of the strain in order to initiate the movement.

Alternatives: Machine Chest Press, Chest Flye, Pec Dec

EXERCISE 16

(a) and (b): Chest Flye

Major muscles used: Pectoralis major

Synergist muscles used: Anterior deltoid, serratus anterior

Main movement: Horizontal adduction of the shoulder

- Make sure the feet are placed firmly on the ground and that the upper arms are parallel to the floor.
- Do not extend the arms fully. Maintain a slight flexion at the elbow joint with the palms facing upwards.
- Bring the weights together in an arcing motion, keeping them in line with the chest.

Awareness points: Avoid fully extending the arms at all times. Lower the weights under control until the upper arms are parallel with the floor and the hands are within peripheral vision. Maintain a normal lumbar curve at all times.

Safety point: As with all exercises, if the hands are in peripheral vision, then the risk of impingement injury at the acromion process (joint between the scapula and clavicle) is reduced.

Alternatives: Chest Press, Pec Dec

EXERCISE 17

(a) and (b): Single-arm Row

Major muscles used: Latissimus dorsi

Synergist muscles used: Brachialis, posterior deltoid

Main movement: Extension of the shoulder/ flexion of the elbow

- Adopt a kneeling position with one leg so that the hip joint of that leg is approximately 90 degrees and the supporting hand is directly below the shoulder.
- Place the supporting leg on the ground slightly away from the bench but at the level of the hip joint.
- Fully extend the arm holding the weight with the palm turned inwards.
- Draw the weight towards the hip joint until the upper arm is parallel with the floor.

Awareness points: Keep the head facing down to maintain neutral cervical spine. Maintain a normal lumbar curve at all times.

Safety point: It is advised to only raise the upper arm until parallel with the floor. If the arm is raised any further than this, then it is the trapezius muscle that is responsible. The latissimus muscle is a much stronger muscle than the trapezius; therefore, if a considerable weight is being used, this could compromise the trapezius leading to strain injury.

Alternatives: Lat Pull-down, Seated Row

EXERCISE 18

(a) and (b): Shoulder Press

Major muscles used: Deltoids (anterior and posterior)

Synergist muscles used: Triceps

Main movement: Abduction of the shoulder/ extension of the elbow

- Stand with feet shoulder-width apart and the spine in neutral position. Ensure upper arms are slightly below parallel position, with hands directly above the elbow joint.
- The palms should be facing forwards and in line with the front of the face.
- Raise the weights in an arcing motion, keeping them in line with the front of the face until the arms are fully extended.

Awareness points: Both hands should remain within peripheral vision at all times. Maintain a normal lumbar curve at all times.

Safety points: Keeping the hands in peripheral vision reduces the risk of impingement injury. Also, to prevent injury to the supraspinatus muscle, a small countermovement bounce should be done at the start of the lift.

Alternatives: Machine Shoulder Press, Lateral Raise, Upright Row

EXERCISE 19

(a) and (b): Lateral Raise

Major muscles used: Deltoids (anterior and posterior)

Synergist muscles used: Trapezius (upper fibres during shoulder elevation)

Main movement: Abduction of the shoulder

- Stand with feet shoulder-width apart and the spine in neutral position. Hang the arms by the sides with a slight bend at the elbow joint so that the weight is slightly forward of the hip joint, palms facing inwards.
- Raise the weights in an abduction motion, keeping them in line and slightly forward of the hip joint until the arms are parallel to the floor.

Awareness points: Both hands should remain within peripheral vision at all times. Maintain a normal lumbar curve at all times. Stop when the upper arms are parallel to the floor.

Safety point: It is advised to stop the movement when the arms are parallel to the floor in order to reduce the risk of impingement with the humerus and acromion process. Also, when going beyond this point it becomes a trapezius exercise; therefore, it is best to perform a specific trapezius exercise, such as a shoulder shrug (see page 52–53).

Alternatives: Shoulder Press, Upright Row

EXERCISE 20

(a) and (b): Upright Row

Major muscles used: Deltoids (anterior and posterior)

Synergist muscles used: Trapezius (upper fibres during shoulder elevation), Brachialis

Main movement: Abduction of the shoulder/ flexion of the elbow/elevation of the shoulder girdle

- Stand with feet shoulder-width apart and the spine in neutral position. Hang the arms to the front of the body with a slight bend at the elbow joint, palms facing inwards.
- Raise the weights in a vertical motion, keeping them in front of the body until the upper arms are parallel to the floor.

Awareness points: Maintain a normal lumbar curve at all times. Stop when the upper arms are parallel to the floor.

Safety point: This is similar to the lateral raise (see page 271) in that when the upper arm goes above parallel to the floor it is the trapezius that becomes the prime mover. However, it is often the case that there is an increased risk of injury due to the extreme angle at the wrist.

Alternatives: Lateral Raise, Shoulder Press

EXERCISE 21

(a) and (b): Triceps Extension

Major muscles used: Triceps

Synergist muscles used: Anconeus

Main movement: Extension of the elbow

- Stand with feet shoulder-width apart and the spine in neutral position. Extend upper arm directly above the head with a 90-degree bend at the elbow, palm facing inwards.
- Extend the arm so that the hand is directly above the shoulder joint.

Awareness points: Maintain a normal lumbar curve at all times. Make sure that the weight remains to the side of the head at all times.

Safety point: There is always a degree of risk when a weight is above the head, so use caution or choose a safer option such as the Triceps Kick-back (see page 274).

Alternatives: Triceps Push, Triceps Kick-back

EXERCISE 22

(a) and (b): Kick-back

Major muscles used: Triceps

Synergist muscles used: Anconeus

Main movement: Extension of the elbow

- Adopt a kneeling position with one leg so that the hip joint of that leg is at approximately 90 degrees and the supporting hand is directly below the shoulder.
- Place the supporting leg on the ground slightly away from the bench but at the level of the hip joint.
- With the palm turned inwards raise the upper arm until it is parallel with the floor and keep a 90-degree angle at the elbow joint.
- Extend the lower arm backwards until it is parallel with the floor.

Awareness points: Keep the head facing down to maintain neutral cervical spine. Maintain a normal lumbar curve at all times. Also, in order to exercise the full range of the triceps, try lowering the upper arm at the end of the movement so that it is below parallel as the triceps crosses the shoulder joint and performs shoulder extension.

Safety points: Try to keep the head facing the floor as there is a tendency to look up and rotate the head to look at the weight, which can cause unnecessary pressure on the cervical region.

Alternatives: Triceps Push, Triceps Extension

EXERCISE 23

(a) and (b): Free-weight Biceps Curl

Major muscles used: Biceps brachii

Synergist muscles used: Brachialis, brachioradialis

Main movement: Flexion of the elbow

- Stand with feet shoulder-width apart and the spine in neutral position. Hang the arms by the sides with palms facing forwards.
- Raise the weights in a line towards the face as if eating.

Awareness points: Maintain a normal lumbar curve at all times. Make sure that the weights do not strike the face and lower them to full extension of the elbow joint.

Safety point: Avoid any twisting motion at the start of the movement as flexion and rotation often lead to tendon problems such as epicondylitis (golfer's or tennis elbow).

Alternative: Biceps Curl Machine

EXERCISE 24

(a) and (b): Squat

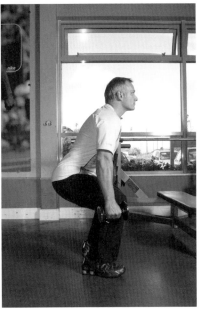

Major muscles used: Quadriceps (vastus lateralis, vastus medialis, vastus intermedius, rectus femoris), hamstrings (biceps femoris, semitendinosus, semimembranosus), gluteus maximus, erector spinae

Synergist muscles used: Some of the muscles above work as synergists depending on the angle of the torso

Main movement: Extension of the spine, hip, knee and ankle

- Stand with feet shoulder-width apart and the spine in neutral position. Hang the arms by the sides with palms facing inwards.
- Bend the hip joint and knee joint as in a sitting motion until the individual is at their full range.

Awareness points: Maintain a normal lumbar curve at all times. The head should drop and raise in a vertical line so that the body does not tilt forward.

Safety point: Always encourage individuals to squat through their full range as limiting the range of motion can lead to weakness (and lack of flexibility) at certain points in the range of the movement.

Alternative: Leg Press

EXERCISE 25

(a) and (b): Chest Press

Major muscles used: Pectoralis major

Synergist muscles used: Anterior deltoid, triceps, serratus anterior

Main movement: Horizontal adduction of the shoulder/elbow extension

- Make sure the feet are placed firmly on the ground and that the seat is at the height where the arms are parallel to the floor.
- The upper arms should be in line with the body.
- Fully extend the arms, keeping the wrists firm.

Awareness points: Maintain a normal lumbar curve at all times. Do not allow the hands to go out of peripheral vision at any time.

Safety points: Most machines allow a starting point where the upper arms are further back than the line of the body. This can place too much strain on the anterior deltoid (as in the free weight version). Set the machine so that the shoulder joint feels as though it is not on stretch.

Alternatives: Free-weight Chest Press, Chest Flye, Pec Dec

EXERCISE 26

(a) and (b): Pec Dec

Major muscles used: Pectoralis major

Synergist muscles used: Anterior deltoid, serratus anterior

Main movement: Horizontal adduction of the shoulder

- Make sure the feet are placed firmly on the ground and that the seat is at the height where the upper arms are parallel to the floor.
- The arms should be in line with the body.
- Bring the arms together under control.

Awareness points: Maintain a normal lumbar curve at all times. Do not allow the hands to go out of peripheral vision at any time.

Safety point: Most pec decs are set up so that the upper arm is laterally rotated in order to place the hands on the pads. This has the effect of wrapping the pectoral tendon over the humerus. In order to avoid this, try doing the exercise with straight arms so that the hands are not on the pads. This will put the pectoral tendon in the right place.

Alternatives: Chest Press, Chest Flye

EXERCISE 27

(a) and (b): Shoulder Press

Major muscles used: Deltoids (anterior and posterior)

Synergist muscles used: Triceps

Main movement: Adduction of the shoulder/extension of the elbow

- Make sure the feet are placed firmly on the ground and the spine is in neutral position.
- Adjust the seat height until the upper arms are slightly below parallel position.
- Raise the arms until they are fully extended.

Awareness points: Both hands should remain within peripheral vision at all times. Maintain a normal lumbar curve at all times.

Safety points: Keeping the hands in peripheral vision reduces the risk of impingement injury. Also, if the upper arms are quite far below parallel at the start position, then injury could occur to the supraspinatus muscle as this would be responsible for initiating the movement.

Alternatives: Free-weight Shoulder Press, Lateral Raise, Upright Row

EXERCISE 28

(a) and (b): Seated Row

Major muscles used: Latissimus dorsi

Synergist muscles used: Brachialis, posterior deltoid

Main movement: Extension of the shoulder/ flexion of the elbow

- Make sure the feet are placed firmly on the floor and the spine is in a neutral position.
- The chest support should be adjusted so that the hands can take a firm grip of the handles with the chest on the support.
- Adjust the seat height so that the arms are roughly parallel to the floor.
- Draw the weight towards the body until the upper arm is parallel with the plane of the body.

Awareness points: Keep the head facing forward to maintain neutral cervical spine. Maintain a normal lumbar curve at all times. Only draw the upper arms back to the plane of the body to avoid undue strain on the trapezius muscle.

Safety point: Limit the movement so that the arms finish parallel to the body. If they pull further back, this will increase the risk of injury to the trapezius as it will be the muscle responsible for this further movement.

Alternatives: Lat Pull-down, Single-arm Row

EXERCISE 29

(a) and (b): Lat Pull-down

Major muscles used: Latissimus dorsi

Synergist muscles used: Brachialis, posterior deltoid

Main movement: Adduction of the shoulder/ flexion of the elbow

- Make sure the feet are placed firmly on the floor and the spine is in a neutral position.
- Adjust the seat height so that the arms are almost at full extension when gripping the handles on the bar.
- Draw the bar vertically down in front of the body until it is roughly in line with the chin level.

Awareness points: Keep the head facing forward to maintain neutral cervical spine. Maintain a normal lumbar curve at all times.

Safety points: Only draw the bar to chin level to avoid undue strain on the rotator cuff muscles as the shoulder would have to internally rotate to go any further. Also, draw the bar to the front of the body to keep the hands in peripheral vision in order to reduce the risk of impingement at the shoulder joints.

Alternatives: Seated Row, Single-arm Row

EXERCISE 30

(a) and (b): Back Extension

Major muscles used: Most of the erector spinae group of muscles

Synergist muscles used: Multifidus and some of the many individual muscles that make up the erector spinae group

Main movement: Extension of the spine

- Make sure the feet are placed firmly on the floor or foot plate and the spine is in neutral position.
- Place the pad across the shoulder level with the torso in a flexed position.
- Extend the back to a position where the spine is in neutral.

Awareness points: Keep the head facing forward to maintain neutral cervical spine. Maintain a normal lumbar curve at all times. Avoid going into extension of the spine.

Safety point: The main role of the erector spinae muscle group is to maintain an upright posture whenever we are in a standing position; therefore, limit the extension (but have a full flexion range) to where the body would be in a vertical position rather than a 'lean back' position.

Alternatives: Free-weight Squat

EXERCISE 31

(a) and (b): Abdominal Crunch

Major muscles used: Rectus abdominis

Synergist muscles used: Hip flexors (iliopsoas), external and internal obliques

Main movement: Flexion of the spine

- Make sure the feet are placed firmly on the foot plate or behind the pads.
- Place the pad across the upper chest or place elbows on the pads.
- Draw the torso towards the knees.

Awareness points: Keep the head facing forward to maintain neutral cervical spine. Maintain a normal lumbar curve at all times.

Safety point: The rectus abdominis is essentially a fast-twitch muscle used for running, jumping and explosive movements; therefore, limit the flexion range or choose an option such as knee lifts.

Alternatives: Knee Lifts, Sit-ups, Crunches

EXERCISE 32

(a) and (b): Triceps Push

Major muscles used: Triceps

Synergist muscles used: Anconeus

Main movement: Extension of the elbow

- Make sure the feet are shoulder-width apart and the spine is in a neutral position. Grip the bar shoulder-width apart so that the upper arms are just forward of the body line, palms facing downwards.
- Extend the upper and lower arm so that the arms are both fully straight.

Awareness points: Maintain a normal lumbar curve at all times.

Safety point: Make sure that there is some shoulder extension in the movement in order to work the full range of the triceps in a functional role.

Alternatives: Triceps Extension, Triceps Kick-back

EXERCISE 33

(a) and (b): Machine Biceps Curl

Major muscles used: Biceps brachii

Synergist muscles used: Brachialis, brachioradialis

Main movement: Flexion of the elbow

- Make sure the feet are shoulder-width apart and the spine is in a neutral position. Grip the handles so that the upper arms are on the pads and the palms face upwards.
- Bring the handles up towards the face until the elbow joints are fully flexed.

Awareness points: Maintain a normal lumbar curve at all times. Keep the upper arms on the pad at all times. Fully extend the arms on the downward phase.

Safety point: Try and position the elbow joint directly in line with the pivot of the machine so that the upper arm follows the arc of the machine handles.

Alternative: Free-weight Biceps Curl

EXERCISE 34

(a) and (b): Seated Adductor

Major muscles used: Adductor longus, brevis and magnus, gracilis, pectinius

Main movement: Adduction of the hip

- Ensure the feet are placed firmly on the foot plates and the pads are on the insides of the knees.
- Use the machine setting to open the legs to a comfortable start position.
- Bring the legs together against the resistance.

Awareness points: Maintain a normal lumbar curve at all times. Keep the knees and the toes pointing directly upwards at all times.

Safety point: The main role of the hip adductors is to stabilise the hip when running and walking; therefore, limit the weight and increase the reps to increase muscular endurance.

Alternatives: Squat, Leg Press, Lunges

EXERCISE 35

(a) and (b): Seated Abductor

Major muscles used: Gluteus minimus and maximus, tensor fascia latae

Synergist muscles used: Sartorius, piriformis

Main movement: Abduction of the hip

- Make sure the feet are placed firmly on the foot plates and the pads are on the outside of the knees.
- Use the machine setting to start with the legs together.
- Open the legs outwards against the resistance.

Awareness points: Maintain a normal lumbar curve at all times. Open the legs to a full range of motion.

Safety point: The main role of the hip adductors is to stabilise the hip when running and walking; therefore, limit the weight and increase the reps to increase muscular endurance.

Alternatives: Squat, Leg Press, Lunges, Multihip Machine

EXERCISE 36

(a) and (b): Leg Extension

Major muscles used: Quadriceps (vastus lateralis, vastus medialis, vastus intermedius, rectus femoris)

Main movement: Extension of the knee

- Place the roller pads just above the ankle joints.
- Use the machine seat-setting to move the seat so that the knee joint is just at the edge of the seat.
- Start with the knees flexed as far as comfortably possible.
- Extend the knees to full range of motion.

Awareness points: Maintain a normal lumbar curve at all times. Keep the knees and the toes pointing directly upwards at all times. Ensure that full extension is achieved.

Safety point: Not going to full extension can result in weakness of the vastus medialis muscle (one of the quads), which only fully contracts in the last few degrees of the movement. If this weakens, it could result in patellar maltracking (where the patella does not run in the groove at the end of the femur) and erosion of the articular cartilage on the underside of the patella.

Alternatives: Squat, Leg Press, Lunges

EXERCISE 37

(a) and (b): Leg Curl

Major muscles used: Hamstrings (biceps femoris, semitendinosus, semimembranosus)

Synergist muscles used: Calf (gastrocnemius and soleus)

Main movement: Flexion of the knee

- Place the roller pads just above the calcaneus or heel bone.
- Use the machine seat-setting to move the seat so that the knee joint is just at the edge of the seat.
- Start with the knees extended as far as comfortably possible.
- Flex the knees to full range of motion.

Awareness points: Maintain a normal lumbar curve at all times. Keep the knees and the toes pointing directly upwards at all times.

Safety points: The main function of the hamstrings is during walking and running when the thigh comes forward (hip flexion) at the same time as the hamstrings contract during knee flexion. If the machine has a pad that comes down on the thighs, try not to use it if possible as this would restrict movement of the thigh, which is what the body is normally used to.

Alternatives: Squat, Leg Press, Lunges

EXERCISE 38

(a) and (b): Leg Press

Major muscles used: Quadriceps (vastus lateralis, vastus medialis, vastus intermedius, rectus femoris), hamstrings (biceps femoris, semitendinosus, semimembranosus), gluteus maximus

Synergist muscles used: Some of the muscles above work as synergists depending on the foot placement

Main movement: Extension of the hip, knee and ankle

- Place the feet about hip-width apart on the foot plate.
- Use the machine seat-setting to move the seat so that the knee joint is flexed to the maximum comfortable position.
- Extend the knees to full range of motion.

Awareness points: Maintain a normal lumbar curve at all times. Keep the knees and the toes in line at all times. Ensure that full extension at the knee joint is achieved.

Safety point: Do not limit the movement to approximately 90 degrees. All individuals should be encouraged to have a full range of movement in order to strengthen at the outer range and help flexibility, which is often lacking.

Alternatives: Squat, Lunges

EXERCISE 39

(a) and (b): Internal Rotation

Major muscles used: Teres major, subscapularis

Synergist muscles used: Latissimus dorsi, pectoralis major, anterior deltoid

Main movement: Internal rotation of the shoulder

- Stand with feet shoulder-width apart and the spine in neutral position. Hold the cable so that the forearm is parallel to the ground and fully externally rotated.
- Bring the forearm across the body.

Awareness points: Maintain a normal lumbar curve at all times. The forearm should remain parallel to the floor throughout the movement. Adjust the tension on the band to suit, if not using a cable.

Safety point: Shoulder stabilisers tend to be weak so encourage lighter weights.

Alternative: Use a flexi-tube or resistance band anchored to a suitable machine at elbow height.

EXERCISE 40

(a) and (b): External Rotation

Major muscles used: Teres minor, infraspinatus

Synergist muscles used: Posterior deltoid

Main movement: External rotation of the shoulder

- Stand with feet shoulder-width apart and the spine in neutral position. Hold the cable so that the forearm is parallel to the ground and fully internally rotated.
- Take the forearm across and away from the body.

Awareness points: Maintain a normal lumbar curve at all times. The forearm should remain parallel to the floor throughout the movement. Adjust the tension on the band to suit, if not using a cable.

Safety point: Shoulder stabilisers tend to be weak so encourage lighter weights.

Alternative: Use a flexi-tube or resistance band anchored to a suitable machine at elbow height

Cardio exercises

The choice of cardio machines is a matter of individual preference: they essentially perform the same function, so any other cardio machine can be used as an alternative. The examples of cardio machines given in this chapter are typical of those used in fitness facilities. It is crucial that all beginners to cardio machines are shown or taught the correct technique prior to performing the exercises themselves.

EXERCISE 41

Treadmill

Foot action: A heel–toe action should be encouraged when walking or jogging, as this will help to absorb the shock of impact. At speeds of around 8mph, the client should be encouraged to use a mid-foot strike, as this will help to eliminate the braking effect.

Arm action: The most efficient way to swing the arms is with a 90-degree angle at the elbows and with the arms swinging close to the side of the body. Try to keep the shoulders relaxed at all times.

Posture: Encourage the client to maintain a neutral spine with only a slight forward lean, which should increase slightly as the treadmill is inclined.

The science: Beginners to this exercise often feel dizzy when the treadmill comes to a stop. This is caused by confusion of signals to the brain. From an individual's very first step, the brain associates each step forward with an increase in size of the images in the distance. As this does not occur when training on a treadmill there is a period of confusion until the individual becomes accustomed to the situation.

Top tip: In the induction, advise beginners to stand still for a few seconds at the end of a session until they feel they are balanced.

EXERCISE 42

Upright Cycle

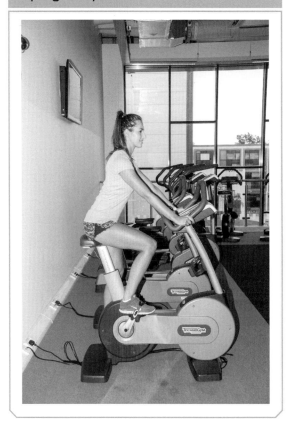

Seat height: As the seat height can affect the range of motion and speed of the legs, it is important to make sure that the seat is in a position that is comfortable for the client but efficient for cycling. With the client on the cycle and the feet flat in the pedals, the knee should have a slight bend at the furthest point of the rotation.

Pedal speed (cadence): Actual pedal speed depends on the preference of the client. Most people prefer to pedal between 50 and 80 rpm, although this can increase during bouts of high intensity.

Posture: Encourage an upright posture with neutral spine at all times.

The science: It is quite common to see people hunched over and resting their elbows on the handles. This is usually down to fatigue of the erector spinae muscles (these are also known as the 'anti-gravity' muscles, as it is their role to keep us upright throughout the day).

Top tip: Encourage individuals to maintain an upright posture for as long as they can and try to reduce the time spent leaning on the handles.

EXERCISE 43

Recumbent Cycle

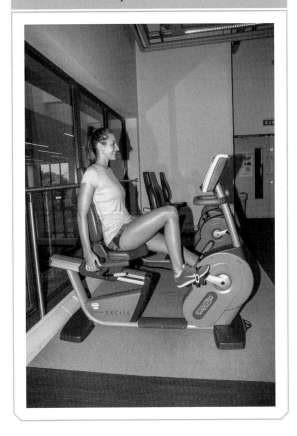

Seat height: As the seat height can affect the range of motion and speed of the legs, it is important to make sure that the seat is in a position that is comfortable for the client but efficient for cycling. With the client on the cycle and the feet flat in the pedals, the knee should have a slight bend at the furthest point of the rotation.

Pedal speed (cadence): Actual pedal speed depends on the preference of the client. Most people prefer to pedal between 50 and 80 rpm, although this can increase during bouts of high intensity.

Posture: Encourage clients not to press their back flat into the seat; try to maintain a neutral spine.

The science: Due to the seat position the pelvis is almost forced into posterior tilt. This has the effect of flattening the lumbar spine, compressing lumbar intervertebral discs, which increases the risk of disc herniation.

Top tip: Encourage individuals to maintain a neutral spine as much as they possibly can.

EXERCISE 44

Stepper

Range of motion: With the foot placed safely and centrally on the step, encourage a full range of motion that is just before the end range of the machine.

Action: As the leg rises during the stepping, the heel of the same leg should rise slightly off the pedal and return to the pedal as the leg goes down.

Speed: Select a speed that is comfortable for the client. As the level on the step machine is increased, the resistance of the pedals will decrease, which means that the client will need to increase the speed.

Posture: Encourage the client to hold the handles just to the side of the body rather than out in front. This will enable the client to maintain an upright posture with neutral spine.

The science: Individuals often complain of having 'tingling' or numb toes as a result of keeping their feet flat on the pedals. With this technique there is no calf contraction, which is one of the main mechanisms responsible for venous return.

Top tip: Always encourage a heel lift as in normal walking.

EXERCISE 45

Cross Trainer

Action: With the foot placed safely and centrally on the step, encourage a smooth running-style action.

Speed: Select a level of resistance that is comfortable for the client. As the level on the machine is increased, the resistance of the pedals will also increase.

Posture: Encourage the client to maintain an upright posture with neutral spine whether holding the fixed or moving handles.

The science: Individuals often complain of having 'tingling' or numb toes as a result of keeping their feet flat on the pedals. With this technique there is no calf contraction, which is one of the main mechanisms responsible for venous return.

Top tip: Always encourage a heel lift as in normal walking.

EXERCISE 46

Rower

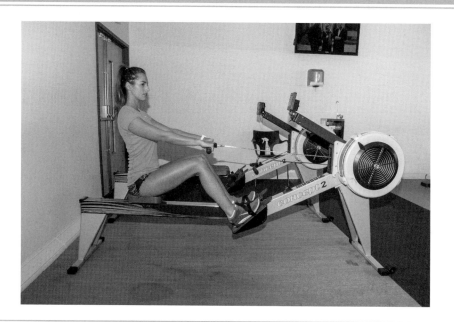

Start position (catch): With the feet secured in the straps and the knees bent, hold the handle with a pronated grip (overhand), with the arms out straight and a slight bend at the elbows. Keep the wrists straight. The back should be in an upright neutral position.

Drive: Initiate the drive phase with the legs pushing out. When the legs are almost at full stretch, pull the handle into the abdomen area.

Recovery: The arms must extend fully before the legs bend to allow the body to come back to the start position. The recovery phase should be twice as long as the drive phase.

Action: With the feet placed safely and centrally on the foot pad, encourage a smooth arm action and controlled pace.

The science: A neutral spine is often difficult to maintain at the end of the drive phase when the legs are at full stretch. This is often due to tight hamstrings keeping the pelvis in posterior tilt and flattening the lumbar spine.

Top tip: Try not to force neutral spine throughout the drive phase and work on hamstring flexibility.

EXERCISE 47

Arm Crank/Ergometer

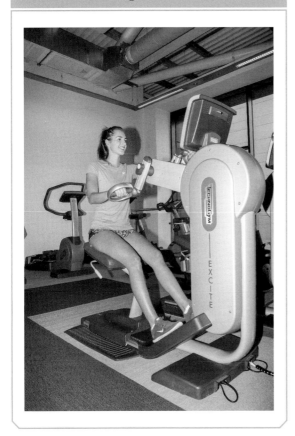

Speed: Select a level of resistance that is comfortable for the client. As the level on the machine is increased, the resistance of the hand pedals will also increase.

Posture: Encourage the client to maintain an upright posture with neutral spine at all times.

The science: As this equipment uses less large muscle groups than other cardio equipment, individuals will find it harder to achieve higher heart rate levels as well as experiencing local muscle fatigue.

Top tip: Do not rely on this piece of equipment as the only machine in a cardio programme or for use in fitness testing unless it is specific to the needs of the client.

Exercise techniques to avoid

Within the health and fitness industry there are many opinions in relation to the technique employed when performing cardio and resistance exercises. The biomechanics of human movement can often help settle certain debates. However, if instructors do not feel they have the necessary experience to draw on published research then it helps to think in simple terms. If a situation arises whereby the instructor is unsure then logical and scientific approaches should be used. Instructors should ask themselves 'would this be typical of human behaviour'? In other words 'is it logical or common sense'? It is then possible to support this logic with a simplified scientific explanation. The following examples might be considered the most common in the health and fitness industry.

ELLIPTICAL TRAINER/STEPPER

Should the client keep their feet flat on the foot plates throughout the movement as in Fig. 15.1a or should they raise their heels as in Fig. 15.1b?

- **The logic bit** If we think about human movement then the answer would be to raise the heel as this occurs during walking, running or going upstairs. The exercise then mimics human movement.

- **The science bit** It is quite common with this type of exercise for clients who maintain flat feet throughout to report a tingling or numbness in the toes. This can be due to lack of venous return

FIG. 15.1

(a) Feet flat

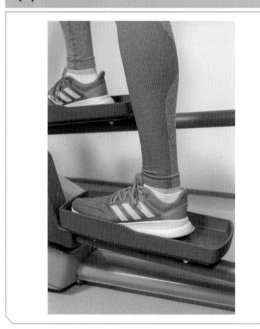

FIG. 15.1

(b) Heel raised

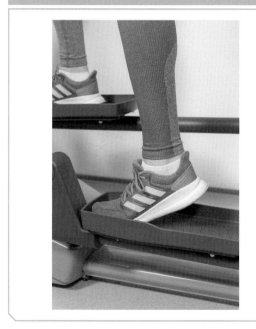

and therefore poor circulation as contraction of the calf muscle (during heel lift – plantarflexion) is one of the main mechanisms for venous return. It can be seen in Fig. 15.1b that with the heel raised, the angle at the ankle (between the tibia and foot) is greater than 90 degrees. This indicates dorsiflexion is taking place and as such calf contraction must be occurring. Always encourage heel lift during this type of exercise.

UPRIGHT AND RECUMBENT CYCLES

Is the recumbent cycle better for back problems? The answer to this common question can be solved by thinking about posture and postural muscles.

● **The logic bit** It is much easier to achieve good posture on an upright cycle as shown in Fig. 15.2a. It can be difficult to

maintain a normal lumbar curve in a reclined posture as in Fig. 15.2b.

● **The science bit** Sitting in a reclined position often results in posterior tilt of the pelvis, which can flatten the lumbar arch, potentially leading to injuries such as herniated discs. Also, in an upright position, many of the core muscles are engaged compared to those in a reclined position. It is quite common that clients might feel the need to lean forwards and support themselves on the handlebars during exercise. This is mainly due to erector spinae muscles being fatigued. These muscles are also known as our 'anti-gravity' muscles as they are designed to keep us in an upright position for most of the day. The instructor should allow a period of rest in this way but then encourage an upright posture again in order to develop muscular endurance in this group of muscles.

FIG. 15.2

(a) Upright cycle posture

FIG. 15.2

(b) Recumbent cycle posture

ROWING

Should clients always sit up straight with good posture throughout the entire drive and recovery phases when rowing? To answer this commonly asked question the trainer should think in terms of hamstring flexibility.

● **The logic bit** Sitting on the floor with outstretched straight legs and leaning forwards with an upright posture is not an instinctive movement. If you have the opportunity to watch a baby or small child then you will see the legs are usually bent and the back will arch.

There are many people who are not capable of sitting in an upright position with natural lumbar curve and reaching their toes as in Fig. 15.3a. In order to reach the toes it would be necessary to arch the back as in Fig. 15.3b.

It is recommended therefore that in such cases the trainer ensures that the client performs hamstring stretches prior to and following the exercise in order to develop hamstring flexibility. For the majority of clients, do not be too strict about posture. By all means encourage and remind clients of good posture but do not force it.

SQUATTING

In fitness environments around the globe you will often hear the phrase 'do not squat below 90 degrees' as shown in Fig. 15.4a.

● **The logic bit** The simple response to this is we should because we can. For many thousands of years humans have foraged for

FIG. 15.3

(a) Upright rowing position

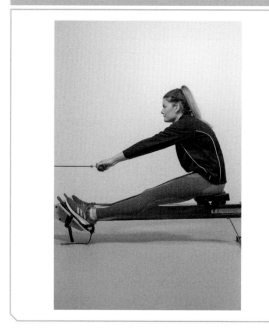

FIG. 15.3

(b) Arched rowing position

FIG. 15.4

(a) Squat above 90 degrees

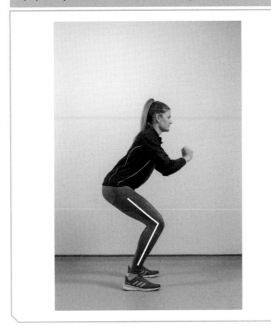

FIG. 15.4

(b) Squat below 90 degrees

food, which requires things to be picked up from the ground. The human body has joints that allow us to squat down below 90 degrees (as in Fig. 15.4b) to be able to do this.

- **The science bit** One of the main reasons that we struggle to squat below 90 degrees as we get older is that we lack the strength and flexibility to do so. The very nature of modern environments limits the degree to which we squat. Since the invention of the chair, we very rarely need to perform squats to any reasonable depth so we lose the ability to do so. It is recommended, therefore, to encourage clients to try to improve their own squat depth and increase flexibility in gastrocnemius and soleus muscles as inflexibility in these muscles can restrict squat depth.

LAT PULL-DOWN

With this particular resistance machine exercise it is common to see individuals pulling the bar behind the head as in Fig. 15.5a as well as pulling the bar to the front as in Fig. 15.5b, but which is more effective?

- **The logic bit** This particular exercise employs the same muscle groups as if an individual was pulling themselves up a tree by a branch or climbing up something like a rock face. In both of these tasks the climber's hands would always be in front of the body and not behind out of view. To mimic this it would require the client to pull the bar in front of the face.

- **The science bit** When the shoulder is in the position as in Fig. 15.5a it is in abduction and external rotation. This is known

FIG. 15.5

(a) Behind the head pull-down

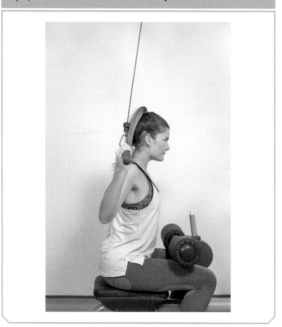

FIG. 15.5

(b) Front pull-down

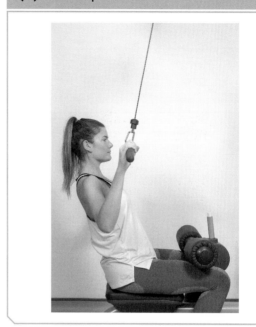

as the 'at-risk' or 'high-5' position and is associated with increased risk of injury, such as impingement or shoulder instability. An easy way to think of this is if the hands can be seen in peripheral vision with the head facing forwards then the shoulder joint should be in a relatively safe position. One of the worst exercises related to this is bench dips (think about the shoulder position).

SHOULDER PRESS – BEHIND THE HEAD

With this free weight or resistance machine exercise there is a perception by some that the rear deltoid muscles are being trained. Is this the case?

• **The logic bit** Think about basic human movement of picking something up to place it at a higher level, such as picking up a heavy log to

place it on top of other logs to build some kind of protective fence. The instinct would be to lift up to chest level then push it up from chest level in front of the face, just as in a clean and press Olympic lift. It would be very unlikely a human would put the log behind the neck to then push it up.

• **The science bit** In order to lift behind the head the humerus must externally rotate as in Fig. 15.6a. This is the high-5 position as mentioned previously, which is associated with increased risk of impingement injury. Also, in the externally rotated position, the anterior deltoid is responsible for the majority of the work as the rear deltoid is almost rotated under the shoulder so that it doesn't contract. If the humerus is brought slightly forward in the sagittal plane (i.e. elbows forward) as in Fig. 15.6b then the hands will be in peripheral vision, which will reduce impingement risk and also employ all the

FIG. 15.6

(a) Behind the head press

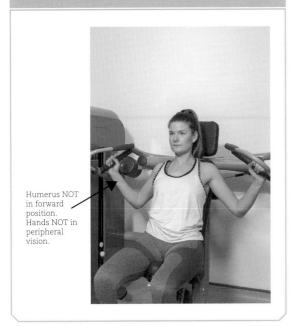

Humerus NOT in forward position. Hands NOT in peripheral vision.

FIG. 15.6

(b) Neutral press

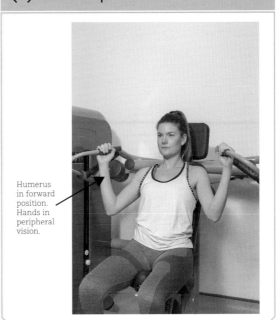

Humerus in forward position. Hands in peripheral vision.

deltoid muscles to do the lifting (known as the neutral press). Simple mechanics!

SHOULDER PRESS – SEATED

This is an exercise that is commonly seen in most fitness facilities but is this more effective than a standing press?

- **The logic bit**   Common sense dictates that as humans we would never be in the position where we would need to lift something above our heads in a seated position. Basic instinct would be to have the weight close to our chest and perform a small countermovement before pushing the weight up so that our leg muscles were involved in the lifting.

- **The science bit**   There are many reasons why we would promote any lifting

from a standing position. Intradiscal pressure (pressure on the discs in the spine known as IDP) is greater in a seated position as opposed to standing. Flexing the knees has also been shown to reduce the IDP during lifting. Also, performing a slight countermovement prior to the lift can help to avoid strain on the supraspinatus muscle (as this muscle initiates shoulder abduction). Research has also shown that there is greater trunk muscle activation in a standing position than in a seated position, therefore strengthening not only deltoids with this exercise but core muscles as well.

UPRIGHT ROWING

This is a very common free weight exercise that is used by beginners and advanced alike; however, is this exercise useful in terms of function?

FIG. 15.7

(a) Seated shoulder press

FIG. 15.7

(b) Standing shoulder press

- **The logic bit** Think about the circumstances in which we would pick up a weight (such as a log or a child). The instinctive way would be to use an underhand grip keeping the weight close to our body. The completely unnatural way would be to take an overhand grip and lift it so that our elbows went out to the side and continue lifting so the weight hit our chin!

- **The science bit** Research tells us that abduction of the humerus greater than 80 degrees can increase the risk of impingement injury. As shown in Fig. 15.8, bringing the bar only to chest level is enough to achieve 80 degrees. As well as being an unnatural movement, this particular exercise does not target any particular muscle as deltoids, supraspinatus, biceps and trapezius are all used.

PREACHER CURLS

Seen in strength and conditioning gyms across the country, this exercise is often employed to increase bicep size. Is this correct?

- **The logic bit** Consider the scenario of a day's hunting and gathering (in the supermarket these days) whereby the spoils of the day needed to be carried home. Imagine bending down, extending the arms out in front and then picking up the spoils using a bicep curl … it's unlikely!

- **The science bit** In a standing biceps curl muscle activation is at its greatest when the weight is furthest from the body as in Fig. 15.9a. This matches the strongest part of the lift (greatest muscle activation) to the point where the weight is the furthest from the body (creating the greatest turning force) as it should do.

FIG. 15.8

Upright row

Humerus at 80°

FIG. 15.9

(a) Biceps curl

Almost the entire range of the lift is done vertically (which is against gravity) therefore effectively creating resistance throughout the entire range. In the Preacher Curl in Fig. 15.9b, when the weight is furthest from the body the arm is almost at full stretch, which is the weakest range for the biceps muscle. Also, almost the entire range of the exercise is done horizontally, which requires almost no effort. Only the first part of the exercise at the extended range requires any vertical movement; however, this is matched to the weakest range of the bicep.

FIG. 15.9

(b) Preacher curl

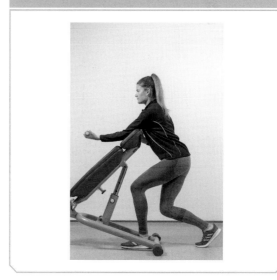

16 Exercise Guidelines for Various Population Groups

OBJECTIVES

After completing this chapter, the reader should be able to:

1. Explain the term 'population groups'.
2. List and explain the benefits of exercise for ante- and postnatal women.
3. List the guidelines for and contraindications to exercise for ante- and postnatal women.
4. List and explain the benefits of exercise for older people.
5. List the guidelines for and contraindications to exercise for older people.
6. Explain the term 'disability'.
7. List typical interaction guidelines for certain disability groups.
8. List and explain the benefits of exercise for younger people.
9. List the guidelines for and contraindications to exercise for younger people.

Introduction

This chapter deals with the background knowledge relating to people who are classified as being in a 'population' group. Within the Professional Standards framework, instructors should be able to list the general exercise advice related to specific groups. Instructors should also be able to describe certain contraindications to exercise.

This chapter builds upon the information in other chapters of this book, regarding the practical application of the theoretical content, to provide the instructor with an understanding of the guidelines for exercise in relation to specific population groups.

Population groups

When prescribing exercise it can be useful to categorise individuals as this can help the instructor determine if they are suitably qualified to do so. For example, instructors need to be suitably qualified to prescribe

TABLE 16.1

RCOG and ACOG exercise recommendations for pregnant women *(Adapted from RCOG and ACOG guidelines.*

	Aerobic training	Strength training
MODE	Walking, cycling and water-based activities are good for this condition	Continue if already active; if not, slow progression from bodyweight to machines/free weights
INTENSITY	RPE level 10–14 60–80% HRmax	Avoid heavy loads Overload by increasing repetitions
DURATION	5–45 minutes per session Increase by 2 minutes per week but only between the 13th and 28th weeks	Perform 1–3 sets of 15–20RM 1–2 minutes' rest between exercises
FREQUENCY	Active person: 3–4 sessions per week up to 14th week 3–5 sessions per week up to 28th week 3 sessions per week after 28th week Non-active person: None before 13th week 3 sessions per week 13th–36th weeks 1–2 sessions per week after 36th week	2–3 sessions per week Encourage other forms of exercise Decrease weight and sets and increase recovery time as pregnancy progresses
PRECAUTIONS	Avoid high-impact activities and excessive repetition Watch for signs of overheating	If no experience prior to pregnancy, do not start Avoid overhead lifts

GENERAL PRECAUTIONS:
Non-active women are advised to seek medical approval BEFORE beginning exercise
If any activity causes pain or discomfort, it should be stopped immediately
Do rectus abdominis check 6–12 weeks after delivery before doing certain abdominal exercises
Be aware of episiotomy and take appropriate steps
Avoid motionless standing, overhead or isometric resistance exercise, loaded forward flexion, rapid change of direction, resisted hip abduction and adduction.

exercise for those with certain long-term health conditions. Instructors may on occasion allow participation from certain population groups as long as it does not become the norm.

ANTENATAL AND POSTNATAL WOMEN

Women from this particular group can participate in group or one-to-one exercise sessions as long as this does not become regular and they meet the following description: 'normal, healthy, adult women experiencing a normal, healthy, singleton pregnancy, or who have had a normal, healthy birth, and who have had previous normal, healthy pregnancies and births'. For obvious ethical reasons research in this area is limited; however, it is generally agreed that in most cases appropriate exercise is safe for both mother and baby. Table 16.1 shows the combined RCOG and ACOG recommended exercise guidelines for pregnant women.

With this population there are certain conditions or factors the instructor should be aware of. Conditions considered serious enough to prevent pregnant women from exercising are known as contraindications to exercise, such as those in Table 16.2.

There are also risks associated with certain conditions deemed not to be serious enough to be termed contraindications. These risks can be minimised by taking appropriate precautions. Table 16.3 shows typical conditions and strategies that can be used to help minimise the associated risk.

Many changes associated with pregnancy persist for several weeks following childbirth. The time considered appropriate to resume or start an exercise programme, however, differs between individuals. Six to eight weeks minimum is usually advised and programmes should be gradually progressive in terms of intensity and duration. An instructor should refer a client to a health professional if she is experiencing any of the following symptoms post birth:

- Stress incontinence or pelvic floor muscle weakness
- 'Dragging' pain or a feeling of heaviness in the lower abdominal or pelvic floor area
- Groin, low back pain or difficulty walking, even if mild and intermittent
- Abdominal muscle weakness, excessive abdominal doming, abdominal muscle separation or softness/sinking at the umbilical midline, umbilical hernia

OLDER PEOPLE

Ageing processes in the body begin around 35–40 years of age. It is not until around the age of 50 that progressive losses in the musculoskeletal, cardiovascular and neuromuscular systems require consideration relating to exercise programmes. In general, the ageing process can result in a 1–2 per cent loss per year in physical capacity in the following:

- Muscular strength
- Power
- Bone density
- Aerobic endurance
- Balance and coordination
- Flexibility and mobility
- Reduced motor learning
- Reduced visual and aural acuity

Instructors who allow over 50s to participate in exercise sessions (albeit not on a regular basis) should be aware of the guidelines in Table 16.4.

In addition, where appropriate, instructors should encourage 50-plus clients to:

- Ensure correct technique
- Take more time during floor to standing

TABLE 16.2

Contraindications and reasons to stop activity for pregnant women
(Adapted from RCOG and ACOG guidelines).

Absolute contraindications to activity:	Relative contraindications to activity:
• Haemodynamically significant heart disease • Restrictive lung disease • Incompetent cervix/cerclage • Multiple gestation at risk of preterm labour • Persistent bleeding in the second and third trimesters • Placenta praevia after 26 weeks • Pre-eclampsia or pregnancy-induced hypertension • Preterm labour (previous/present) • Preterm rupture of membranes	• Severe anaemia (haemoglobin less than 100g/l) • Unevaluated maternal cardiac arrhythmia • Chronic bronchitis • Poorly controlled type 1 diabetes • Extreme morbid obesity (BMI >40) • Extreme underweight (BMI <12) • Extremely sedentary lifestyle • Intrauterine growth restriction in current pregnancy • Poorly controlled hypertension/pre-eclampsia • Orthopaedic limitations • Poorly controlled thyroid disease • Poorly controlled seizure disorder • Heavy smoker (more than 20 cigarettes/day)

Reasons to stop activity

• Excessive shortness of breath • Chest pain or palpitations • Presyncope or dizziness • Painful uterine contractions or preterm labour • Calf pain or swelling • Leakage of amniotic fluid • Vaginal bleeding • Excessive fatigue • Abdominal pain, particularly in back or pubic area	• Pelvic girdle pain • Reduced foetal movement • Dyspnoea before exertion • Headache or visual disturbance • Muscle weakness • Sudden calf pain or swelling in the ankles, hands or face • Insufficient weight gain (less than 1kg per month) during last two trimesters

TABLE 16.3

Risk-minimising strategies

Condition and potential risk	Minimising strategy
Hormonal and postural changes can result in joint misalignment, muscle imbalance, motor skill decline and hypermobility. These changes become more significant as pregnancy progresses.	Avoid repetitive high-impact, excessive or aggressive movements for at least 6 months after birth. Post birth reinforce good posture, joint alignment and stabilisation.
Post birth there is increased risk of air embolism, thrombosis and haemorrhage.	Do not begin exercising post birth without permission of a health care professional (usually at the post-partum 6–8-week check).
While childbearing, posture is forward flexed with shoulder girdle protraction and thoracic kyphosis. This can result in long, weak upper back extensors, and short, tight pectoral muscles and neck and shoulder pain are common.	Focus on strengthening extensors (erector spinae, trapezius and rhomboids) and stretching pectorals.
Lack of abdominal support from transversus abdominis and pelvic floor muscles.	Avoid using sit-up, crunch or oblique-type exercises for at least 12 months. Stabilisation exercises such as abdominal bracing are recommended.

- Simplify exercises that the client struggles with
- Avoid extreme spinal flexion

For certain population groups there are contraindications and key safety guidelines for working with older participants as can be seen in Table 16.5.

DISABLED PEOPLE

A person can be regarded as having a disability if he/she has a physical or mental impairment that has a substantial and long-term adverse effect on their ability to carry out normal day-to-day activities. According to the English Federation of Disability Sport there are between 8 and 12 million people in the UK with some

TABLE 16.4

ACSM and AHA exercise recommendations for older adults

	Recommendation
1	All people over the age of 50 should complete a pre-exercise health-screening questionnaire (PAR-Q+ or AHA/ACSM) to establish whether they are asymptomatic and ready to participate or whether they should seek further medical assessment prior to participating in an exercise programme.
2	Increase the duration of the warm-up; i.e. longer than that recommended for adults under the age of 50 years. Clients can be empowered to take responsibility for this such as by walking to the session or by coming early and warming up before the session.
3	Carry out joint mobilisation exercises prior to the main activity, such as shoulder rolls or spine rotation and side bends.
4	Prescribe a more gradually tapered cool-down after the main cardiovascular activity. Clients should be advised to do this by taking responsibility for themselves, for example, by keeping going for a few minutes after the rest of the class have stopped and/or are changing to the next activity.
5	Ensure clients stay within prescribed training zones. The use of RPE is recommended for this. Educate the client on the use of RPE.

degree of disability or impairment as defined as Disabled under the Disability Discrimination Act 1995 (DDA). Unfortunately, disabled people can experience barriers to accessing sufficient physical exercise due to psychological, physical or social reasons. Regular physical activity can help disabled clients in the same way as for non-disabled clients, and may also reduce the risk of gaining additional disabling conditions, improve the ability to perform activities of daily living that might previously have been difficult, and maintain or even improve independence.

The DDA states that it is unlawful to refuse to serve a disabled person, provide a lower standard of service, or offer a less favourable service to a disabled person. Service providers must make 'reasonable adjustments' to their facilities and services so that they are accessible to disabled people. Exemption from the DDA is justified for the following reasons:

- If by meeting the needs of the disabled person the health and safety of any person, including the disabled person, is endangered.

TABLE 16.5

Absolute and relative contraindications to exercise testing *(Adapted from the American College of Cardiology and American Heart Association exercise testing guidelines).*

Absolute Contraindications	Relative Contraindications
Acute myocardial infarction (within 2 days)	Left main coronary stenosis
Unstable angina	Moderate stenotic valvular heart disease
Uncontrolled cardiac arrhythmias causing symptoms of hemodynamic compromise	Known electrolyte abnormalities (hypokalemia, hypomagnesemia)
Uncontrolled symptomatic heart failure	Mental or physical impairment leading to inability to exercise adequately
Acute aortic dissection	Severe arterial hypertension; resting diastolic BP >110mmHg and/or resting systolic BP >200mmHg
Suspected or known dissecting aneurysm	Tachyarrhythmias or bradyarrhythmias
Acute myocarditis or pericarditis	Hypertrophic cardiomyopathy and other forms of outflow tract obstruction
Acute pulmonary embolus or pulmonary infarction	High-degree atrioventricular block

- If by serving the needs of the disabled person the service provider is unable to serve others (not including a delay or inconvenience to others).
- If the disabled person is unable to enter into a legally enforceable agreement or give informed consent.
- If providing a service to disabled people on the same terms as to other people means that it would not be possible to offer the service at all, or if a higher charge would have to be made to others.

For those who are supervising activities it is often not the ability to adapt the activity that is the problem. Problems normally arise when interacting with individuals with disabilities. Even though the list of disabilities is extensive, there are certain ones that instructors might come across that can be grouped together for the purpose of simplicity. These areas include

TABLE 16.6

Interaction guidelines for disability groups

Disability group	Interaction guideline
Speech impairment	Be patient when communicating. Don't speak for the person. Allow them to answer in their own time. Sometimes short questions (or closed questions as they are known) that require short answers or a nod or shake of the head are recommended. Never pretend to understand if you do not. Just be honest.
Wheelchair users	Any equipment a person may use, such as a wheelchair, is part of that person's personal space. Don't physically interact with an individual's body or equipment unless you're asked to do so or you ask first. When speaking with someone in a wheelchair, try to be at their eye level without kneeling. If a person transfers out of a wheelchair, to a car for example, leave the wheelchair within easy reach. Remind people to drink regularly as overheating often occurs. Encourage changing seat position often as circulation may be poor.
Hearing impairment	To get attention, tap the person on the shoulder or wave your hand in front of them. Find out if the person prefers sign language, gesturing, writing or speaking. Look directly at the person and speak clearly and slowly. Speak in a normal tone of voice. Try to talk when background noise is low. Face the sun if you are outside and try to have light on your face if you are inside. Written notes can often help. Do not talk while writing. If you have trouble understanding, just let the person know.

TABLE 16.6 (CONTINUED)

Interaction guidelines for disability groups

Vision impairment	Always identify yourself and others when meeting someone with vision impairment. It helps to tell the person that the conversation is finished and that you are moving. When you give help, allow the person to take your arm so you can lead. When offering a seat, place the person's hand on the back or arm of the seat. Try to be consistent in each session with things like leaving equipment in the same place. Use 'clock clues' to help orient in the room. Use large print when writing or giving notes.
Learning disability	Be patient and make sure you understand. Use precise and simple language. Try to use words that relate to things around you that you both can see. Try to give the same information in different ways. If you are not sure about the response, repeat the question in a different way. Give exact step-by-step instructions. Ask the person if they prefer information in a verbal or written format. Give constant reminders such as drink and use sun cream regularly.

wheelchair use; hearing, speech or vision impairment; and learning disability and the use of simple guidelines related to each of these areas can be helpful (see Table 16.6).

YOUNG PEOPLE

For the purpose of exercise instruction young people can be classed as aged 14 to 17 years.

It is essential that instructors who work with this age group on a more than occasional basis understand fully the physiological and psychological implications of working with adolescents, to enable them to work safely and effectively within these environments. It is widely acknowledged that muscular strength and endurance exercise can be beneficial to a person's growth and development. The

TABLE 16.7

General guidelines for cardio and resistance training for adolescents

Guidelines for cardiovascular training in adolescents:

1	Interval training should be the main focus for cardiovascular sessions as it provides variety, which may impact on enthusiasm, motivation and confidence.
2	Use the Rate of Perceived Exertion (RPE) scale rather than heart rate to measure intensity. RPE requires the young person to pay particular attention to how tired they feel, how much effort it is taking and how much physical stress they are under.
3	It is recommended to start to educate the participant in the use of heart rate charts alongside the use of RPE until full physical maturity has been reached.
4	PAR-Q+ screening should be adapted for adolescents. The PAR-Q+ should also be signed by their parent or guardian, if they are under the age of 16, to allow access into the gym prior to their first session.

Guidelines for strength training in adolescents:

1	The instructor should only supervise if they hold an appropriate qualification.
2	It is important not to impose adult training regimes on young people and recognise the developmental age of the adolescent; not just their chronological age.
3	Progression in repetitions and sets should only occur when the adolescents are ready both physically and mentally.

British Medical Association state that a young person's fitness routine should include activities that are aerobic or endurance based in order to improve the cardiovascular and cardiorespiratory systems. The instructor should be aware that exercise can impact young people both physiologically and psychologically and therefore should understand the associated considerations.

Physiological safety considerations:

- A gym environment is typically designed for adult frames; therefore, equipment should only be used that is suitable for the size of the young person.
- Focus on variety within a session to avoid excessive or repetitive training.
- Limit the amount of high-impact exercise.

Psychological safety considerations:

- Use simple language to avoid confusion.
- Implement gym rules and boundaries from the onset.
- Be mindful of negative psychological changes such as depression, social issues (such

TABLE 16.8

BASES resistance training guidelines for young people

Frequency	2–3 times a week to develop strength. Rest between sessions: 48 hours' recovery for heavier training sessions
Intensity	Lighter resistance (15–20 repetitions) Moderate resistance (10–15 repetitions) Heavier resistance (6–10 repetitions)
Time	Sets: begin with single sets and progress to 3–4 sets Rest (between sets): will vary depending on training goals. Circuit resistance training should be encouraged to maximise cardiovascular benefits
Type	Promote muscle balance and joint stability by using a whole-body approach and working all major muscles Avoid too much eccentric muscle work

as violence), smoking and drugs, eating disorders and even over-training.

There is a range of guidelines for cardio and resistance exercises for young people depending on the source of the literature. Table 16.7 gives a general overview adapted from several sources.

More specific guidelines have been published by the British Association of Sport and Exercise Sciences (BASES) for muscular training with children and young people as shown in Table 16.8.

The instructor should note that with adolescents training within a gym environment the instructor is in 'loco parentis' and it is their responsibility to ensure the individuals are using the correct and suitable equipment according to their stature and mental capacity. In legal terms this is known as duty of care.

Example Question Answers

1 THE SKELETAL SYSTEM

1.1   The ulna bone is an example of which type of bone?
    a) long bone

1.2   The patella is an example of which type of bone?
    d) sesamoid bone

1.3   The pelvis is an example of which type of bone?
    c) flat bone

1.4   What is the name for the area near the end of a long bone where growth occurs?
    b) epiphysis

1.5   Which two regions of the spine are secondary curves?
    c) lumbar and cervical

1.6   In which region of the spine are the bones fused?
    d) sacrum

1.7   Tendons attach to a layer of tissue covering a bone. What is this covering called?
    d) periostium

1.8   Cells in the bone that are responsible for bone-building are called what?
    b) osteoblast cells

1.9   Cells in the bone that are responsible for breaking down bone are called what?
    c) osteoclast cells

1.10 In terms of postural deviation, an excessive primary curve of the thoracic region of the spine is usually referred to by what name?
    d) kyphosis

1.11 In terms of postural deviation, an excessive secondary curve of the lumbar region of the spine is usually referred to by what name?

    a) lordosis

1.12 In terms of postural deviation, twisting of the spine is usually referred to by what name?

    b) scoliosis

2 JOINTS

2.1 The tibia and the fibula make what type of joint?

    a) fixed

2.2 The facet joints of the transverse processes of the spine make what type of joint?

    a) cartilaginous

2.3 The tibia and the femur make what type of joint?

    c) synovial

2.4 The pubis symphysis is what type of joint?

    b) cartilaginous

2.5 Which of the following is classed as a hinge joint?

    c) elbow

2.6 Which two movements are available at a saddle joint?

    b) flexion, extension, adduction and abduction

2.7 Which of the following make a joint?

    c) femur and pelvis

2.8 Which of the following make a joint?

    b) humerus and scapula

2.9 Which of the following make a joint?

    a) metacarpals and phalanges

2.10 Which of the following make a joint?

a) tarsals and tibia

2.11 Which of the following make a gliding joint?

c) bones of the carpals

2.12 Which of the following make a pivot joint?

b) atlas and axis

3 THE MUSCULAR SYSTEM

3.1 What is the main fuel of type I fibres?

a) fat and oxygen

3.2 What is the main fuel of type IIb fibres?

c) glucose

3.3 Which type of muscle can be found in the digestive system?

d) smooth

3.4 Which type of muscle can be found in the heart?

b) cardiac

3.5 In muscle contraction, which hormone is released from the end motor plate and crosses the synaptic gap?

b) acetylcholine

3.6 Which term is used to describe a muscle under tension where the origin and insertion move away from each other?

c) eccentric

3.7 Which term is used to describe a muscle under tension where the origin and insertion move closer together?

b) concentric

3.8 What is the name given to a muscle when performing the role of stabilising a joint?

d) fixator

3.9 What is the name given to a muscle when performing the role of assisting the agonist muscle?

c) synergist

3.10 What is the name given to a muscle when performing the main action?

a) agonist

3.11 Which exercise is associated with the sagittal plane?

d) leg extension

3.12 Which exercise is associated with the frontal or coronal plane?

c) pull down

4 CARTILAGE, LIGAMENTS AND TENDONS

4.1 What type of cartilage can be described as a thin, tough, shiny, bluey-white membrane?

c) articular

4.2 What type of cartilage can be described as bundles of fibres that provide flexible support?

b) elastic

4.3 What type of cartilage can be described as a thick, strong and spongy shock-absorber?

a) fibro

4.4 What is fibro cartilage mainly made up of?

b) collagen

4.5 Which is a ligament of the knee?

c) lateral collateral

4.6 Which is a ligament of the shoulder?

c) coracohumeral

4.7 Which is a ligament of the hip?

a) ischiofemoral

4.8 Which is a ligament of the ankle?

   b) calcaneotibial

4.9 Which type of tissue connects bone to bone?

   c) ligament

4.10 Which type of tissue connects muscle to bone?

   b) tendon

4.11 What is the name of the fibro cartilage in the knee joint?

   d) meniscus

4.12 Which type of tissue does the statement 'allows wanted but prevents unwanted movement' relate to?

   c) ligament

5   NERVOUS AND ENDOCRINE SYSTEMS

5.1 Glands are responsible for secreting what into the bloodstream?

   c) hormones

5.2 Nerve endings are responsible for secreting what?

   a) neurotransmitters

5.3 Nerves that lead away from the central nervous system are known as what?

   b) motor or efferent

5.4 Nerves that lead back to the central nervous system are known as what?

   a) sensory or afferent

5.5 Which of the following receptors sense position?

   a) proprioceptors

5.6 Which of the following receptors sense pain?

   c) nociceptors

5.7 Which of the following receptors sense temperature?

   d) thermoreceptors

5.8   Which of the following receptors sense chemical composition?

b) chemoreceptors

5.9   Catecholamines and corticosteroids are secreted by which gland?

d) adrenals

5.10 Tyrosine-based hormones that regulate metabolism are secreted by which gland?

b) thyroid

5.11 Glucagon is secreted by which gland?

c) pancreas

5.12 Testosterone and oestrogen are secreted by which gland?

d) testes and ovaries

6   ENERGY SYSTEMS

6.1   When a phosphate molecule is split from ATP, what does it leave?

d) ADP

6.2   What is the main process that occurs within mitochondria?

b) production of ATP in the presence of oxygen

6.3   Anaerobic glycolysis is …

b) breaking down glucose without the presence of oxygen

6.4   Aerobic glycolysis is …

a) breaking down glucose in the presence of oxygen

6.5   Which of the following is given off as a by-product of aerobic glycolysis?

d) carbon dioxide and water

6.6   Which of the following is given off as a by-product of anaerobic glycolysis?

c) lactic acid

6.7   Which of the following is produced as a result of incomplete breakdown of fat due to lack of available carbohydrate?

c) ketones

6.8   Which energy system contributes the most (in percentage terms) at the start of exercise?

   c) ATP–PC system

6.9   Which energy system contributes the least (in percentage terms) at the start of exercise?

   d) aerobic (fat)

6.10   Which energy system contributes the most (in percentage terms) in short sprint events such as the 100 metres?

   c) ATP–PC system

6.11   Which energy system contributes the most (in percentage terms) in events such as the 800 metres?

   b) aerobic glycolysis

6.12   Which energy system contributes the most (in percentage terms) in events such as a long distance run?

   b) aerobic (fat)

7   THE HEART AND THE CIRCULATORY SYSTEM

7.1   The heart muscle is divided into left and right sides by what?

   d) septum

7.2   The heart muscle is entirely covered by a layer of fibrous tissue known as what?

   a) pericardium

7.3   The term 'entry hall' relates to which structure in the heart?

   c) atrium

7.4   The mitral valve is otherwise known as the what?

   c) bi-cuspid

7.5   The sino-atrial node can be found in which chamber of the heart?

   a) right atrium

7.6   The aortic valve can be found leading from which chamber of the heart?

   d) left ventricle

7.7 The amount of blood pumped out of the ventricles each beat is known as what?
c) stroke volume

7.8 The amount of blood pumped out of the ventricles each beat, multiplied by the heart rate in beats per minute, is known as what?
b) cardiac output

7.9 The amount of blood left in the ventricles after each beat is known as what?
a) end diastolic volume

7.10 Which of the following protect the body against foreign bodies?
a) white blood cells

7.11 Which of the following help in blood clotting?
b) platelets

7.12 Blood pressure is greatest in which vessel?
c) aorta

8 THE RESPIRATORY SYSTEM

8.1 What structures lead directly into the alveoli?
a) bronchioles

8.2 The double membrane surrounding the lungs is known as what?
b) pleura

8.3 The passage of oxygen and carbon dioxide in and out of the alveoli is known as what?
a) gaseous exchange

8.4 What is the percentage of oxygen in the air that is inspired?
c) 21

8.5 The amount of air left in the lungs after a breath out is known as what?
c) residual volume

8.6 The maximum amount of air breathed out of the lungs after a maximum breath in is known as what?
d) vital capacity

8.7 Which of the following gases stimulates breathing when blood levels reach a certain point?

b) carbon dioxide

8.8 The amount of air taken into the lungs during a normal breath is called what?

b) tidal volume

8.9 Smoking is thought to be one of the main causes of what?

a) chronic bronchitis

8.10 Inflammation of the alveoli is otherwise known as what?

c) pneumonia

8.11 Normal expiration is brought about as a result of what effect?

d) elastic recoil

8.12 Which is the main muscle involved in forced expiration?

d) transversus abdominis

9 CORE STABILITY

9.1 Which of the following properties relates to stabilising muscles?

d) postural, endurance, tonic, slow-twitch

9.2 Which of the following properties relates to mobilising muscles?

c) short-term, explosive, phasic, fast-twitch

9.3 Which of the following can be considered to be predominantly stabilising muscles for the core?

b) multifidus, transversus abdominis, pelvic floor

9.4 Which of the following can be considered to be predominantly mobilising muscles for the core?

c) erector spinae, external oblique, rectus abdominis

9.5 Which of the following can be considered to be a predominantly stabilising muscle for the hip joint?

d) gluteus medius

9.6 Which of the following can be considered to be predominantly a mobilising muscle for the hip joint?

b) gluteus maximus

9.7 When local muscles contract to compress the 'fluid ball' in the abdomen it is known as what?

b) intra-abdominal pressure

9.8 An increase in the tension of the connective tissues in the spinal region is known as what?

d) thoraco-lumbar fascia gain

9.9 Research has suggested that what percentage of maximum contraction is sufficient to create sufficient intra-abdominal pressure to stabilise the spine?

d) 30

9.10 What best relates to the statement *'when there is minimal force placed on the spine and the structures that surround it such as tendons, cartilage and ligaments'*?

b) neutral zone

9.11 True or false? Normal screening procedures should be carried out prior to prescribing core stabilisation exercises but those with back problems should be excluded.

True

9.12 The length of time, number of repetitions and frequency of practice of conscious contraction required to develop subconscious contraction control of the transversus abdominis can take up to how long?

d) a few months

10   COMPONENTS AND PRINCIPLES OF FITNESS

10.1 The ACSM defines what as *'an ability to perform daily activities with vigour and the demonstration of traits and capacities that are associated with a low risk of premature development of hypokinetic diseases'*?

c) health related physical fitness

10.2 The World Health Organization defines what as *'a state of complete physical, mental and social well-being and not merely the absence of disease or infirmity'*?

a) wellness

10.3 Cardiovascular endurance is also known as what?

b) aerobic capacity

10.4 $mlO_2.kg^{-1}min^{-1}$ is a measurement of what?

c) VO_2 max

10.5 What are the benefits of regular cardiovascular training?

a) increased HDL, increased exercise threshold, decreased heart rate for given intensity

10.6 What is the term used to define an increase in muscle cross-section?

c) hypertrophy

10.7 What is the term used to define a decrease in muscle cross-section?

b) atrophy

10.8 What are the benefits of regular resistance training?

a) increased glucose tolerance, increased bone mass, increased resting metabolic rate

10.9 Strength gains in the first few weeks of a resistance training programme are usually due to what?

d) neural changes

10.10 What type of stretching involves the contraction of the agonist to elicit a stretch in the antagonist?

b) dynamic

10.11 Which of the following formulae can be used to calculate BMI?

b) weight/height^2

10.12 In relation to BMI, what figure is classed as obese?

b) over 30

11 SCREENING FOR EXERCISE AND SAFETY ISSUES

11.1 The PAR-Q+ is a screening questionnaire used to identify conditions prior to encouraging exercise at:

c) a light to moderate intensity

11.2 The PAR-Q+ is a screening questionnaire which is valid for what period of time?

d) 12 months

11.3 True or false? The PAR-Q+ is a confidential document.

True

11.4 Which of the following best describes the term 'myocardial ischaemia'?

b) obstruction of blood flow to the heart

11.5 Which of the following best describes the term 'dyspnoea'?

d) abnormally uncomfortable awareness of breathing

11.6 Which of the following best describes the term 'tachycardia'?

d) resting heart rate over 100bpm

11.7 Which of the following best describes the term 'bradycardia'?

c) resting heart rate below 60bpm

11.8 Which of the following best describes the term 'oedema'?

a) swelling usually caused with fluid build up

11.9 Which of the following best describes the term 'claudication'?

c) pain in the lower extremities

11.10 Which of the following best describes the term 'orthopnoea'?

c) shortness of breath lying flat

11.11 The Health and Safety at Work Act (HSWA) 1974 outlines which of the following as roles of the instructor?

c) both A and B

11.12 True or false? The Health and Safety (First Aid) Regulations 1981 states that employers provide adequate equipment and facilities to enable first aid to be carried out on employees but not necessarily customers using the facility.

True

12 BEHAVIOURAL CHANGE AND GOAL SETTING

12.1 The Stages of Change Model follows what type of pattern?

b) cyclical

12.2 Approximately what percentage of all individuals will experience relapse back to the contemplation or pre-contemplation stage?

c) 15%

12.3 True or false? Cognitive processes are usually adopted by individuals in the early stages of the Stages of Change Model from not thinking about exercise to the action of taking up exercise.

True

12.4 True or false? Behavioural processes are usually adopted by individuals in the later stages of the Stages of Change Model.

True

12.5 What is the following a definition of? *'The internal mechanisms and external stimuli that arouse and direct our behaviour'.*

d) motivation

12.6 Which term is used to describe when an individual is motivated to exercise by factors such as enjoyment, fun or self-satisfaction?

a) intrinsic motivation

12.7 When a skill is broken down into manageable units that the subject can focus on, it is otherwise known as what type of goal?

c) process

12.8 The World Health Organization suggests an average daily intake of carbohydrate, fat and protein for the general population should be made up of which of the following?

b) 30% fat, 10–15% protein, 55–60% carbohydrates

12.9 Which of the following vitamins is considered to be important for promoting calcium absorption from food?

c) D

12.10 Which of the following vitamins is considered to be important for producing blood-clotting proteins?

b) K

12.11 Which of the following minerals is considered to be important for brain and nerve function?

b) potassium

12.12 Which of the following minerals is considered to be important for the regulation of body water content and nerve function?

a) sodium

13 COMPONENTS AND INDUCTION OF AN EXERCISE SESSION

13.1 According to research what is considered to be the main factor in muscular injury prevention?

b) muscle temperature

13.2 In terms of cardiovascular training at the end of the warm-up the heart rate should be at what level?

c) that required for the cardiovascular session to follow

13.3 In relation to cardio training zones, what range of heart range maximum is the 'weight management zone'?

b) 60–70%

13.4 In relation to cardio training zones, what range of heart range maximum is the 'aerobic zone'?

c) 70–80%

13.5 Which of the following are considered to be the main benefits of cardiovascular training?

d) increased fat metabolism, increased glycogen stores, increased aerobic and anaerobic enzymes, increased number and size of mitochondria

13.6 What type of training is otherwise known as 'speed play'?

d) fartlek

13.7 Which cycle of periodisation is usually associated with a 7-day period?

b) microcycle

13.8 Which cycle of periodisation is usually associated with a period of a few weeks?

c) mesocycle

13.9 Which cycle of periodisation is usually associated with a 12-month period?

d) macrocycle

13.10 The ACSM guidelines for stretching suggest holding the stretch for what period of time?

b) 15–30 seconds

13.11 The acronym IDEA refers to what?

a) induction for cardiovascular machines

13.12 Which of the following cardiovascular machines is normally associated with higher impact?

c) treadmill

14   MONITORING EXERCISE INTENSITY

14.1 What is the formula for predicted maximum heart rate?

c) 220 – age

14.2 True or false? Predicted maximum heart rate can have an error of up to plus or minus 12 beats per minute.

True

14.3 True or false? A graded maximum heart rate test should be used on all individuals to find their maximum heart rate.

False

14.4 What is the predicted maximum heart rate for a 29-year-old person?

b) 191 bpm

14.5 What is 70 per cent of predicted maximum heart rate for a 40-year-old person?

c) 126 bpm

14.6 What is 80% of predicted maximum heart rate for a 20-year-old person?

a) 160 bpm

14.7 What is 55% of predicted maximum heart rate for a 31-year-old person (round up)?

d) 104 bpm

14.8 What is the equivalent value of 2 MET?

c) 7 $mlO_2.kg^{-1}min^{-1}$

14.9 What is the equivalent value of 1 MET?

a) 1.0 $kcal.kg^{-1}hr^{1}$

14.10 How many kilocalories would an 80kg person expend in 30 minutes doing an exercise valued at 5 METs?

d) 400

14.11 How many kilocalories would a 60kg person expend in 2 hours and 30 minutes doing an exercise valued at 4 METs?

c) 600

14.12 Which of the following statements is most accurate in regards to the definition of 12RM?

d) A weight that can be lifted 12 times and not 13 times

Index